Keep Sparkling!
Saya Rasmussen

CW01305056

# Doing It With Bling On

## BATTLING BREAST CANCER WITH STYLE

Sonja Rasmussen

authorHOUSE®

*AuthorHouse™ UK Ltd.*
*500 Avebury Boulevard*
*Central Milton Keynes, MK9 2BE*
*www.authorhouse.co.uk*
*Phone: 08001974150*

*© 2010 Sonja Rasmussen. All rights reserved.*

*No part of this book may be reproduced, stored in a retrieval system, or transmitted by any means without the written permission of the author.*

*First published by AuthorHouse 4/28/2010*

*ISBN: 978-1-4490-8622-0 (sc)*

*This book is printed on acid-free paper.*

"I was just thinking … you don't need to read about other people's cancer battles….

You can write your own."

Chris Dunhill, friend

And I did!

To Matthew and Emma with love...
this is mummy's story. I know as you grow up
you will move on and forget this year ever happened. But it did
happen, it shaped your childhood,
and you gave me the reason to run towards
the finishing line, face up to the sun,
laughing all the way. You are wonderful,
you are my life and you made my journey
back to health worthwhile.... my story is for you.

# Foreward

**By Prof S D Heys, Consultant Breast Surgeon**
Chair in Applied Medicine, Aberdeen University BMedBiol, MBChB, MD, PhD, FRCS(Eng), FRCS(Ed), FRCS(Glas), FHEA

As a surgeon and specialist in breast cancer for twenty years, I have read many books and written many articles about breast cancer, its causes and how to treat it. We all know how common it is, how it has become more common in recent years and that 45,000 women are diagnosed with breast cancer each year. Now, 1 in 9 women will develop breast cancer, and for every 100 women with breast cancer there is one man diagnosed. We all know that the chances of beating breast cancer are getting better every year and now almost 80% of women will be alive and well five years later.

We have also heard about the treatment such as chemotherapy, radiotherapy and hormone therapy, and we know what effects the treatment can have on us as well as the cancer. The new advances are there for us to see every day on television, and in newspapers and magazines. But the stark reality always at the back of our minds is that not everyone beats breast cancer. I am sure it has affected each of us in some way - either through family, friends, acquaintances or people we work with or meet in our daily lives.

But these are just statistics. What is important - no, what is THE most important thing, is the impact that breast cancer, or a cancer of any kind, has on that person, their family and their friends. How a person deals with their cancer during a journey which I think is one of the most difficult and traumatic experiences that will ever be faced is always unique and very personal.

To make a diagnosis of breast cancer, and to give this news to any patient is a life changing event. Life can, and will, never be the same again. Things change in an instant. What was important one minute prior to those words "....it is cancer...", is no longer important, and may even be completely irrelevant. There is a dawning, a realisation, perhaps immediately or certainly very quickly, that many things around us that were taken for granted are actually the things in life that really matter.

When I was asked to write a foreword for this book by Sonja, I readily agreed. As her surgeon and one of the large team who was looking after her medical care, I wanted to help. I really wasn't sure what she was going to write about, but having got to know her, I knew from the way that she had dealt with everything during her encounter with cancer that this would be an honest account of what happened. It would be personal and it would give an insight that we as doctors and nurses and all who will read this book would be privileged to share with her. I knew that this book would be something special.

I have read stories of how people with cancers are affected and I am sure you have too. But this book is different as you will find out when you read it.

So, it is a story about fear, and the fear for Sonja was of breast cancer and all that that entailed for her. It is a story of how one person had to face up to that fear, how they looked it straight in the eye and how they set about not only conquering the fear for themselves but then, armed with a team of friends, turned that fear on itself and joined in the fight against cancer with their activities.

This is a book that you will not be able to put down. I couldn't until I had finished and that was not because Sonja has promised that I will be portrayed by George Clooney when the film is made!

It will make you sad, it will make you happy, it will make you think and reflect. What if....what if this was me....? How would I face up to what lies ahead and what might or might not happen?

This story will inspire you. It has inspired us, the doctors and nurses who look after patients with cancer. This is pure inspiration on paper!

As Sonja says in the book............"this is how it is".

# Introduction

**The sun shines on the righteous –
Text from Lisa, Bling Fling committee**

It seemed to me that there had never been so much rain fall in one day than on the Saturday before the first ever Bling Fling.

As the heavens opened and the torrents poured through, I consoled myself with the thought that my friends and I had done all we could. The hours we had spent organising the Tiaras and Trainers Charity Walk and Party, which would over the next few months raise tens of thousands of pounds for Breast Cancer Research, could achieve no more. Only a power far larger than ours could ensure the weather was in place for the day...

Twenty-four hours later, and a transformation had occurred. On a day as beautiful and sunny as Aberdeen can occasionally muster, the Bling Fling was born and with it, a celebration of fun and friendship and all the other strengths that women are blessed with.

Forgive me, I haven't introduced myself. My name is Sonja Rasmussen, I am 40 years old, and I have fought and won my battle with Breast Cancer.

At the time I was diagnosed, I was also a theatre critic, journalist and drama teacher, mum to Matthew and Emma, wife to Graham, daughter to Mary and Eric Rasmussen, sister, sister-in-law and auntie in an extended and loving family ... you get the general idea, I had much to live for...

I know that I am one of the lucky ones... I have met and connected with many people over the last year who have also been fighting cancer in its many guises. Some are still with us. Others, sadly, are not and the world is a far poorer place without them.

Whatever direction their battle took them, however, these people were all in their own way, special.... brave, inspirational, focussed and steadfast, courageous in the face of adversity and a tower of strength in the midst of their own battle.

Everything about cancer is random. You develop it, you don't, you recover from it, you don't. There is no rhyme or reason as to those who survive, or those who fall victim to its evil clutches...

From day one of my cancer diagnosis, I did not look for reason or blame, for these feelings, in my eyes, were too destructive. Instead, I chose to look for the positives - the good times that kept me going – family and friends around me, my children who kept everything normal, the laughs, the cinema trips during the day (how decadent did that feel?), the endless and supportive phone calls across the miles, the texts giving words of encouragement or praise, and yes, even computer social networking sites which gave a link to the outside world and reminded me that others were living their lives and going through their own crisis not too far away.

When the Bling Fling took place on May 17th, 2009, it marked an end to my treatment and raised an incredible £73,000 for three Aberdeen charities – including Breast Cancer Research at Aberdeen Royal Infirmary, under the leadership of Professor Steven Heys, the man who brought me through my personal cancer journey, and has become a friend and ally over the past year.

He jokes about being played by George Clooney in the film of my life – I haven't quite decided who would play me yet – and I have agreed, so George, if you are out there and reading this, sometime in the future you may have to get to know one very clever man by the name of 'the Prof', a man to whom I owe my life.

In the months after the Bling Fling, everywhere I went I heard about it, people asked about it, gave money to it – and the final total was breath-taking and life-changing for the charities involved. But perhaps more importantly for me, it fulfilled another, more personal aim - it celebrated life and friendship, giving me the chance to thank all those special friends and family who were my inspiration for every smile and laugh shared along the difficult road we had travelled.

All those mentioned in the following story have joined me on my journey, and there are many others who have cheered me on from the sidelines – and for that I will always be grateful. A fight against breast cancer is not one that can be faced alone … and a veritable army helped in mine.

Now back to the beginning… to the last days of summer, before the news that would make my world implode, with my loved ones standing by to catch the pieces and mend them together again, one by one…

This I wish for you...
For every storm a rainbow,
For every tear, a smile
For every care, a promise
And a blessing in each trial...

For every problem life sends
A faithful friend to share
For every sigh a sweet song
And an answer to your prayer...

Card from Beverley, Stephen and Katie Walker, Singapore

# Chapter 1

**"Have you called the doctor yet...? Please go and do it"**
Erica, younger sister

'WHAT if it is – you know (at this point we couldn't bring ourselves to say the C-word)?'

'Oh come on, it won't be. '

As my fingers went self-consciously to the lump, I was disappointed to find it was still there.

Each time my hands were drawn to the spot I had discovered a small, but very noticeable lump as I was showering a couple of days before, I felt disappointed. Surely it was going to go away – spots did that. Appeared – usually just before a night out – and gone again within a few days. Not so, it seemed, this one.

I was newly 40. Well, fit, active, and always thinking of my diet. Detoxing was a pastime of mine. I was strangely drawn to blueberries, consuming them with a passion while investing great trust in them that they would be shifting the toxins, keeping me safe from the C-word. See, again I can't say it.

But there it was, underneath my skin. A small, hard lump that didn't move when I pushed it, didn't shy away from my touch. It just sat, quietly indignant, willing me to do something about it.

"Call the doctor."

"No, not yet... Let me wait a few days – see if it goes away first." My voice dropped letting the doubt creep in.

What if? What if?

"Call the doctor." My sister Erica has always been the go-getter. The fixer. The meeting organiser, report writer, the one who does. She pushed me to phone. Thank God…

That first visit to the surgery was, as I recall, pretty uneventful. After suggesting I had 'lumpy breasts anyway' – (I'm sure a compliment in some parts of the world? – that's the way I took it anyway) – the GP referred me to the hospital.

Huh? How did that happen? Why was I not like those other people – the ones who get lumps all the time? Who said that they were cysts and assured me mine would be the same.

Absolutely typical of me. Being different is what I strive for, individuality, creativity, refusing to follow the crowd. Different is a good thing. Is it not?

**Hi Sonj. Graham mentioned you had to go to hospital yesterday. Hope all is okay? – Text from Gav, friend**

The hospital? Oh yes, the hospital. Well I went – thanks to my ever supportive parents, who rather than watching me worrying myself (and them) sick, offered to pay for a first appointment at the private hospital, jumping the queue which I had landed at the bottom of. Don't ask me why… age? Seemed I wasn't the only one to think I was untouchable by the C-word.

Anyway, in the somewhat more salubrious surroundings of the Albyn Hospital, and accompanied by my partially sighted mum and her beautiful guide dog Campbell, who seems to sense when a girl is down and needs a bit of tender loving care Labrador style - I had the first of many tests, 'the lump' put at the mercy of clamps, cameras, scanners and needles, as they tried to get their hands on the cells in question.

'Like chasing a pea around a dinner plate,' I was told.

And then … oh god no … the results … deep breaths… don't cry… Campbell put his head into my lap and looked deeply and reassuringly into my eyes.

Of course, I couldn't meet the eyes of the man who could give me the answers. My mind was everywhere other than in the room at that particular time, and however kind Professor Heys was – and, in my eyes, he is truly the kindest and most sensitive doctor I have ever encountered – what he said next was the last thing I had ever expected or wanted to hear.

"I'm seriously concerned about this lump Sonja."

Breathe …

"I'm going to treat you at the hospital. "

Oh no.

"You'll be in my care for the next five years."

Keep it together Sonja.

"Do you want to take these leaflets home to read and prepare yourself – some people don't want to know at this stage. It's entirely up to you …"

Oh shit … he thinks I've got breast cancer. Doesn't he know how old I am, the children I have, the life I lead? …. Oh no … no… no… please let him be wrong.

Outwards, do you know what I said? – "Guess that makes me trendy. Kylie Minogue has had it, why shouldn't I?"

While inside my head, screaming from the very depth of me "I'm too young to die, I'm too young to die."

Coming home that first night, I was a changed woman. Sure I looked the same – long hair down my back, vintage waistcoat, my obligatory bit of bling round my neck.

But inside, I was different. I had crossed that one-way bridge to become a breast cancer sufferer, a journey from which I would never return.

I could look back and see the trouble-free past I had come from, but I'd never again be able to cross to that place where my health was taken for granted and my future was secure.

From now on, I would be a survivor, brave, inspirational … but never just Sonja.

**Hi. Hope you are okay and managed to get some sleep. Thinking about you all the time XX Text from Fiona, childhood friend**

Sleep? Sleep? When you have so much to read, to digest, to take into your already traumatised mind… sleep seemed the last thing my mind wanted to do.

Instead, I would think … and dwell … and worry … and think some more.

I did read the leaflets, books, anything that would allow me a window on other people's battles. All digested in the half-light of early morning. Mentally preparing myself while the world slept for the battle of my life...

**I have thought about you so much. It must all be terrifying but try and keep calm. Lots of love Fiona XX - Text**

# Chapter 2

## Lots and lots of love XX

My dad is a businessman. Still in charge of a family firm at 65, he loves every minute of his working life.

He's also a family man, generous of spirit and fun to be with.

I love him for his strength, for his ability to make things right and to find fun in the worst situation.

So when he told me 'It'll be all right. You'll get through this,' you know what? I believed him. I looked into those kind experienced eyes, just as I have done throughout my life, and I knew it was going to be okay …

It's a funny feeling. Suddenly being a child again, needing a parent to hug, kiss it better, make it go away.

In my dad's way, I guess that's exactly what he did … gave me the chance to talk without interruption or judgement, and made me believe I was up to this, I could get through it … then stood back and let me do it in my own way.

Mum has always been the tower of strength in our family, a person admired by all who encounter her, a teacher, inspirer and friend to many.

She is my first port of call in any storm, and she is the one who was with me at the beginning. Mum shared that initial shock, the leap into the unknown, the sleepless nights as we both struggled to cope with the news.

As the days went on, I found my closest relationships became the most difficult. Each time I was with mum, I cried. I stopped coping, our relationship reverted to a childhood one, mother and child, each reassuring one another and sapping each other's ability to cope at the same time.

She turned to me for reassurance – "Can I tell this group of friends... maybe they should know?" and the more she struggled to come to terms with it, the more I backed off.

I needed space to do this my way. Mum needed to be sure she was playing it as I wanted her to. Finally, I told her; 'Tell those friends who you depend on, just as I have done.

"I need you to be able to speak to someone else about your fears and worries. I'm struggling with it myself. I've got to stay strong for my children. I need you to cry with other people and stay strong for me."

In my irrational way, I see now, I blamed her ... for not being able to make it good, make it fair, sort it out for me.

And she regretted that she was struggling with those things too... That's what mums are for after all. The whole world knows it.

The only thing is, there are some things even the How To Be A Good Mum Handbook doesn't sort out for you. And coping with your 40-year-old daughter getting breast cancer is one of those things ...

In the months since that first diagnosis, mum and I have talked, cried, laughed, let each other be and shaped a new, more grown-up relationship. Mondays established themselves as our day together – trawling charity shops for clothing gems became a new shared passion, or on chemotherapy weeks, walking Campbell in the gorgeous woodland around Aberdeenshire, always followed by tea and chat. And of course, the best medicine of all, no matter how old you are, lots and lots of cuddles.

I grew up as the eldest of a family of four – until I was 18-months old, I was younger sister to the first-born Rasmussen baby Craig, who died just before his third birthday, a tragedy for my parents which, of course, had a huge bearing on their reaction to their eldest daughter getting breast cancer.

I have two sisters – Heidi, who works in the National Health Service and is the most practical person I know (especially in a medical crisis) and Erica who lives in Aberdeen, and was able to be around for me throughout this story.

My youngest brother Keith is the calming influence on his big sisters – as a child he christened us 'the Uglies'. He's the only one (apart from my dad) who still uses my childhood nickname Soggs. Even when we worked together at our family firm, he'd use it in front of customers... and not quite understand why I'd get embarrassed. As far as Keith is concerned, a bit of gentle teasing never hurt anyone. He is right and that's exactly how he played it... Always the same, always with a one-liner at the ready, and I love him for it.

As the only boy in a family of girls, he's pretty good at chat too – couldn't get a word in edgeways most of the time if I'm honest – but is always there with a cup of tea on the brew at the welcoming Aberdeenshire farmhouse he shares with his wife Claire and ever growing family. Their third Rasmussen boy arrived just after I was diagnosed, guaranteeing plenty of cuddles in the first few months, and someone to compare hairstyles with as my mop started to return after chemotherapy had wreaked its havoc.

Heidi is the only one of us who really flew the family nest, settling with her husband Simon in the south of England in her early twenties. They have two children of similar age to ours, who spend many school holidays in Aberdeen with their cousins – building relationships as special and long-lasting as ours have been despite the years and miles between us.

My diagnosis corresponded almost perfectly with Heidi returning to work as an Occupational Therapist after a ten year break from the National Health Service. Although a plane trip away, however, she stayed involved in every way possible, always there on the end of a phone, helping by answering my questions where she could, advising me where to look for answers within the NHS, providing the voice of reason when I was having a stressful moment and advising me at all times 'not to be a superhero – take the drugs they give you, rest, don't do too much... take time to smell the roses along the way'. In fact, Heidi is so good at giving advice, you'd think she was the older sister - and at times I think it's always been that way.

And then my youngest sister Erica - well, she was there whenever and however she could be…

She lives in Aberdeen with her husband Ewan, who runs a family business and is constantly adding to the steading they have shared for almost 20 years. They have three children, Erica is lecturing full-time as well as studying for a PhD, and it did not seem possible she would have had the time to dedicate to me over the next six months, But dedicate it she did – listening, advising, speaking for me if I was struggling for words at appointments, asking questions when I couldn't think of them, being there.

And for our children … she provided the bridge between them and my breast cancer. She talked them through it, let them cry, listened and answered their questions, took them into her family for weekends and did everything – and I mean everything – possible to help.

How anyone gets through a crisis without an Erica on hand, I'll never know.

My husband Graham, as the eldest of four boys, is a strong, quiet, hard-working type.

I've always thought him the rock that can cope with my theatrical, at times manic personality. I seemed to have done enough talking, crying, laughing, you name it, for both of us during our 12 year marriage.

The night of my cancer diagnosis changed him too. His kingdom was shattered. His wife, strong and confident, mother and homemaker, was gone. In her place was a little girl, lost, scared and clinging to her family for support.

It's not easy for me to remember how Graham coped during those first few days. I know he was struggling, I know he talked more candidly to my sister than he had ever done before. And I know he told my friends more about how he was feeling than he told me.

We protected each other, I guess. I turned to friends, my parents, my siblings - anyone whom I felt could cope with what I was going through.

Meanwhile, Graham also dealt with it in the way with which he felt most comfortable – he tackled 'the problem' as he saw it from a very practical (and of course very male) point of view, and set about the task of providing for his family.

Graham had recently started a new business, having been made redundant from his job as television cameraman and editor a few months earlier. I knew that starting out on his own, after 21 years of financial security at a firm he loved, was a big deal for him – and of course, for us as a family. If we couldn't afford to pay the bills, it would impact on our lifestyle, our home, the children's future. Let's face it... the problems of my breast cancer would have far wider implications if the cash ran out.

And so we decided that the best way forward was for Graham to concentrate on establishing his company, allowing me the time to get better. Over the coming months, Graham worked from home, looking after the children when I wasn't well enough or was busy with hospital appointments, giving me the chance to go through treatment in my own way while growing his business in the credit crunch climate.

I asked other friends and family members to join me for appointments, giving Graham space and time to work, and in some ways, this was the perfect solution all round.

In others, however, I see now that it excluded him and allowed our paths to separate for a time, bringing problems and resentments to the surface later, when we started re-emerging at the end of this traumatic year.

All in all, however, I love him for what he has done and achieved on our behalf, and thank him for giving me, and the children, the time and support we needed to get through this.

As I've said often, and I'm sure will say again, you can't plan your battle against cancer. The shock of diagnosis changed my life and the lives of those around me, and in some ways, things will never be the same again.

The advice given by my nurse to 'take one day at a time' seemed trite and somewhat flippant in the beginning. But, you know what. It's true. The journey is long and you can't go it alone. There are many bridges to cross and hurdles to encounter, but none are insurmountable.

Those decisions I made in that first week were the knee jerk reactions of shock. Time brings clarity ... and purpose. And what's more, it heals.

You just have to let it happen.

## Chapter 3

**Shit, shit and double shit! Text from Sandy, Friend XX**

Okay, Sandy is my friend along the road. The night I came home from the first tests, I knew I had to go and see her.

I needed her sense of fun, her Zimbabwean take on life, her ability to put her foot in it and make me laugh all at the same time.

I needed to cry, to laugh at myself crying, to laugh at her crying at me, to laugh.

And we did just that. Drank peppermint tea, chatted as if nothing was wrong… chatted as if everything was wrong and nothing would ever be right again… and laughed at the hopelessness of it all.

I remember Sandy saying: 'God, I'm such a klutz. Why do I keep saying the wrong things …'

'Sandy you're saying all the right things', I told her. "You're making me laugh … just keep doing that'.

Laughter is what keeps us going when the world is collapsing around us I find…

**Just wondering how it's all going. So worried about you. Hope you are ok and the news is not too bad. Lots of love Fiona X**

Fiona has been my friend since we were four years old and I love her to bits. Although she has lived in London since she was

19, we are as close now as we have ever been, and I am so glad she happened to be visiting Aberdeen the night before I went to the hospital for the first time.

It was Fiona that first put the idea of cancer in my head ... for some reason, she says now, she had a feeling it wasn't going to be 'just a cyst', 'a blocked pore' or any of the other reasons I had conjured up.

She was worried, and although she had returned home to London, and her husband and three children by the time I got the news, she called, she listened to me, she spoke sense, she cried, she let me cry and she gave me confidence from afar that I could get through this.

Many times throughout this journey she has told me she loves me, and with a 36-year friendship behind us, I know she means it. What a privilege to hear your friend say such things. For a moment – and not for the first time over the following months - I realised how lucky I was.

**Waiting is shit, but we are all waiting with you and remember I am a witch and you will come out on top..." Text from Nicola, friend X**

Telling close friends over the first few weeks was tough. Tough on me, tough on them ... but in a strange way, one of the most bonding experiences a friendship can ever go through.

The people I chose to confide in respected my wish to keep it quiet until I knew what was happening (and more importantly until I had told the children), and for that I will always be truly grateful.

The endless cups of tea, cuddles, concern, help and hope kept me going over the first few weeks. Each time I told someone, registered their shock, and then talked them through their worries for me, the burden got a little lighter and easier to handle.

Until I felt that my breast cancer was affecting everyone. All who knew were involved and beside me, sharing the battle with me. You need an army to fight an enemy, and my little group of friends were my personal soldiers in the early days, and remained shoulder to shoulder with me throughout my cancer fight.

> **Was thinking about you the day.**
> **Keep strong as I'm sure you will be.**
> **Text from Gav, friend XX**

Strong? What makes us strong? Everyone finds strength in different things, but for me, strength is found in projects, in staying focussed, in being in control.

I wanted life to go on as normal in those early days. To forget I had breast cancer. To do what other women of my age and stage were doing. To have fun. And that's exactly what we did.

> **You were amazing this weekend. So strong ... what a star X**
> **Skerry, sister-in-law**

There was a weekend in Loch Lomond planned for my father-in-law's 70th birthday. A gathering of the Read clan as it were – eight children, ten adults, all ready to have fun. And then there was me, harbouring a secret as huge as I could bear inside my head, taking over my very core, enveloping every thought and rendering me useless at the process of socialising – which is a necessity on a family birthday.

At first, I thought I should bail out. I wanted to run and hide, stay inside my head for a weekend, dwell on the uselessness of it all, cry.

But, of course, there were the children – and the fact that nobody but Graham knew. I needed to go. I needed to have a bit of fun for their sake – and, as it turned out, mine too. And so I cushioned myself by sharing my huge secret. I told Skerry.

Skerry is my sister-in-law. She is married to Graham's brother Michael, has two little boys and runs a successful business. Something of a high flyer by all accounts... She's also the sister-in-law who wasn't pregnant at the time, or visiting from Switzerland. She is a strong, caring individual, who says all the right things and knows how to cope in every situation. She is bright, breezy, the centre of every conversation – many of which she has started - and a terrific actress... adding up to the perfect choice of secret-bearer!

> **Hope you're bearing up darlin'. Sending positive thoughts your way. Am here if you need anything at all ... Skerry XX**

When I told her, she hugged me, cried (as I did), then with strength enough for the two of us, shouldered the burden and took it on herself to protect me over the weekend and the coming weeks, shielding me if I needed comfort, allowing me space for my thoughts and giving Graham and I time to talk – never an easy thing when there is a houseful of family to contend with.

We had a fantastic weekend – well, at least, I had a fantastic weekend. Graham remembers it being the worst of his life. Where I had been dealing with the shock and worry for days before, I needed a release – and chatting about ordinary things with people who didn't yet know what was going on provided exactly that.

For Graham meanwhile, the shock wave hit over those two days in the Highland Lodge. After focussing on work and avoiding the issues at the outset, his feelings started to surface when he had time to think – hard-hitting and deep-rooted hurt and anxieties that he would take months to really come to terms with, if indeed ever.

I, however, managed to keep my own mood more buoyant than I thought possible by distracting myself with the younger children in the family (who didn't notice if I had a tear in my eye), and dancing to the Mamma Mia soundtrack while drinking red wine to my heart's content - purely medicinal of course, and far more appetising than any medicine to follow thereafter.

It all seemed surreal, to be honest, and the world of breast cancer seemed a lifetime away from this happy gathering of family and friends. I could forget, and live a little. And that's exactly what I needed and did.

Before the weekend ended, I let my other sisters-in-law into my inner circle of 'those who knew' – Rachel, who is married to Graham's brother David, and was seven-months pregnant with her third child, and Emma, married to Stephen, second son in the Read family, and living in Switzerland with their two young children.

My parents-in-law I told later, once the dust had settled from the celebrations. The months leading up to my father-in-law's 70th birthday were filled with happy planning and travel arrangements. Bringing together a family of four boys – one of them from overseas – along with their busy wives, and eight young grandchildren is no mean feat. I wasn't going to be the one to throw a spanner in the works of the meticulously planned weekend by making any big shock announcement.

Besides, I was aware that Millie and Ed are worriers by nature, and as a couple have had their own health issues over the years which they have dealt with in a way quite different from that which my naturally gregarious personality will allow. Their problems are handled quietly, almost insularly, away from the hustle and bustle of family life, and because they're not my parents, I wasn't sure how to tell them or indeed how they would cope with the news of my having breast cancer.

When I did finally come clean, once the excitement of the birthday had subsided, they were of course terribly upset, called my parents to offer their support, and worried about the outcome for me. They were the first to articulate the fear that I might die of this, leaving the children to go on without me at such a young age. I can't say I wasn't thinking those things too – of course anyone who is told they have cancer must come to terms with their mortality at some point thereafter, but as a self-preservation tactic, I chose not to dwell on those thoughts.

They also realised that Graham and I had spent the whole weekend pretending that nothing was going on – they were both inspired by our bravery, and upset that we felt we couldn't share the news with them or that they were so wrapped up in the fun of the weekend that they hadn't noticed what we were going through.

Actually, I like to think that the fact we chose this particular path was of mutual benefit. We were all able to enjoy a weekend of peaceful, almost normal life, preparing ourselves for the months ahead when, as they say, we would hit the rapids and cling on for dear life ... the calm before the storm.

**"Hi Sonja. Thinking of you and Graham every minute. You have been absolutely amazing this weekend, so strong. What an inspiration. I can't put into words what I want to say but we love you and Graham so much." Text from Rachel, sister-in-law**

From Skerry, the day after the Bling Fling, May 17 2009

Dearest Sonja

Just a note to say a really huge well done on the Bling Fling - the scale of what you and your committee achieved in such a short timescale is quite beyond belief and truly inspiring to say the least.

You must be so delighted at how amazing all the pink t-shirts looked both at the warm up (she was good!) and as we all walked into the sunny distance and then back to the delights of the amazing ambiance created at the Winter Gardens ... creating some really lovely memories for every participant for sure.

When I think about that weekend in Loch Lomond and how far you've come since then, never looking anything less than fabulous every time I've seen you, and how amazingly positive you've been throughout, I'm really lost for words.... a rare occurrence indeed.

You are the real deal Sonja, living life to the full and trail blazing a path ahead in spite of a crisis... a Pepsi Max queen indeed and I was privileged to learn at the Bling Fling what an inspiration you are to so many as well as me ... you are a gift, you make a difference.....

Keep blinging darlin'....
All my love
Skerry Read, Team Electra

# Chapter 4

**What a bloody nightmare. Poor you. – Text from Gavin**

Gavin is one of my oldest friends. I met him and his wife Susan over 20 years ago while performing in the university's Student Charities' Show, and over the last two decades we have become the best and closest of friends. Their daughter Ailsa was my flower girl, and took on the role of niece before I had any real ones to add to my now ever-growing collection.

Gavin takes no nonsense from me. He will never be fobbed off with 'I'm fine', and has the knack of getting to the root of my problems, listening, forcing me into vocalising my thoughts and making me laugh even when it seems there's nothing much to laugh at. He totally summed it up with this text.

The first two weeks were a nightmare.

I knew I had breast cancer. The Prof had ascertained that much on that first night at the private hospital.

But they still had to find out what kind – invasive, non-invasive, size, what it responded to, if it had spread. All this before they could decide on treatment.

And that took time. As they said before, finding the lump in the breast tissue of someone my age was tricky. It was mobile, moved whenever they tried to stick a needle in. Can't say I'm surprised, judging by the size of those needles, I would do the same!

They did the first needle test … or core biopsy as they called it in the medical world … and I waited for results. And finally, after a week on tenterhooks, the phone rang.

The news? They'd have to do it again. And so the nightmare began.

**Presumably they are still keeping you waiting for further news. Thinking about you so much. Fiona X**

Looking back, that waiting game during the first few weeks was the worst part of this incredible journey. And part of the problem in those early days was the lack of anyone apparently fighting my corner.

I was assigned a Breast Cancer Care nurse at my first appointment, who kicked off on the wrong foot with me when she told my partially sighted mum, who had requested some Breast Cancer Care information leaflets on Cd so that she too could listen and learn from them, that she wouldn't like them because 'they were read in a posh voice.' Okay, I could rise above that one, but it was her lack of commitment to my case that started to irk with me over the next few weeks.

She was older and in the twilight years of her nursing career, while I was vulnerable and starting out on a journey into the unknown, and I can see now that we just didn't hit it off – in fact, I'd go so far as to coin a phrase my group of friends often laugh at as being a strange and rather quaint expression – 'she just wasn't my cup of tea'.

Actually I don't know what 'my cup of tea' is – Earl Grey, Peppermint, Ginger, Apple and Cinnamon, Tetley. You name it – any cup of tea will do in this lady's crisis. And when it comes to people, I'm very much the same. My friends are all very individual and varied, with their own strengths and weaknesses, each bringing something different to my life. But collectively, they are strong, reliable, loyal women and men – everything, in fact that I looked for in a nurse and at this point was not finding.

'We'll get the results back in a couple of days. I'll call you Tuesday morning at 8.30am', I remember her saying. Right, that's quite specific, I thought, and hung onto that day and time in my head, waiting by the phone on the assigned date for the call to come through.

Each minute, then hour that passed, became more agonising for me – looking for those promised calls felt like some kind of cruel torture, another form of pain being inflicted on top of the dicing with death game I was already playing.

When I eventually decided enough was enough, and called her myself, it seemed I spurred her into action, reminding her that she had to get onto my case, and the answers were found in a couple of hours...

How this compounded my stress, I can't tell you. The frustrations of playing a waiting game at that stage would have been enough to send me over the edge, had I not been supported as I was by the most fantastic group of family and friends cheering me on, persuading me to pick up the phone, encouraging my strength when I was all set to lie down and give up.

And finally, after two weeks of worry and sleepless nights, which pushed me as low as such constant stress tends to do, the call came in...

The bad news – they'd have to do one final, ultra sound guided core biopsy which would lead them straight to the area in question, guaranteeing they harvest the rogue cells. The good news – it would take place tomorrow.

**Hi. Hope all goes well. Will be thinking of you a lot. Think you are amazing and gorgeous so be strong! Keep me posted! X Text from Lesley**

Lesley is one of my Bling Girls. Without having breast cancer, I doubt I'd ever have discovered her strengths, if I'm honest.

She is a mum of three children, wife and homemaker – always with a cup of tea at the ready for me, and an open door policy for all those lucky enough to be her friends.

At this stage, she was the one who joined me at the hospital, holding my handbag as I stripped off, dressed and stripped off again for what seemed like endless mammograms and needle tests.

Sympathising with my frustration, sharing a cup of tea in the hospital canteen as we waited for yet another appointment, and laughing – and Lesley can laugh – as we paced the corridors from clinic to clinic.

Lesley has a laugh that is instantly recognisable – I have traced her in a crowded disco by the fantastic sound of happiness that emanates from her readily and often. What's more, her laughter envelopes everyone and everything around her, giving even the worst situation a far brighter appeal.

**One hurdle down. Well done you.
Not sure I'd let a Mr Bean lookalike near me? Ailsa**

**Imagine if he'd looked like George Clooney! Nicola**

Yes, okay the consultant radiographer looked like Mr Bean, but thankfully that's where the similarity ended. He was professional, calm and totally trustworthy, and I felt at last, I was going to get some answers ...

"This must have been an awful shock for you... is there anything you don't understand about what we're doing ... tell us what you want to know and we'll give you as much information as we can at this stage."

Whoa, hold the bus...rewind a little. He's asking ME if I want to know anything... at last I had found someone in this huge and faceless hospital community who would answer my questions. Someone who would speak to me, treat me as a person, let me in on the inner world of the medical profession.

And so I spoke, and I asked, and I discovered that I did indeed have breast cancer, that they needed to get tissue from the lump so that they could treat it, and that it was invasive, fast-growing and had already broken through some of my breast tissue.

From that moment on, I surrounded myself with the people who saw me, Sonja. Not just a patient. Sonja - who had a life, children, husband, family and friends – all who loved me. I had to get through this for their sakes - and mine – and I needed people on side who understood that.

In the next few weeks, this would give me the confidence to choose my personal medical team. I realised there was nothing set in stone – except, of course, the fact I had cancer. Everything else was open to negotiation, and I was the one at the reins.

# Chapter 5

**Have you got your appointment yet? Hope Emma has a fab birthday. Skerry X**

I am lucky enough to have been blessed with two beautiful children – Matthew and Emma.

Matthew was nine when I was diagnosed with breast cancer. Handsome, blonde and full of energy, I have often been told he will break many hearts. I've no doubt about it – he's my son after all.

Emma is my baby – pretty, delicate, with a gorgeous, gentle nature and a beautiful all-encompassing smile.

On the day my breast cancer became part of their lives, Emma was celebrating her seventh birthday with a fairy tea party after school.

As I put the finishing touches to the games, party bags and fairy décor – planning a seven-year-old's party is a time-consuming affair, especially when you're distracting yourself from the thought of having breast cancer - the phone rang.

The oncologist had my results and wanted to see me. Could I come in right away, say in half an hour?

Leaving Graham with his instructions – a five-minute run-down on hosting the best ever fairy party (a task which, by all accounts, I had prepared him for and teased him about constantly over the last few weeks – I seemed to know somehow that this scenario was likely - and, of course, he was perfectly capable of and happy to carry out) – and accompanied by Erica with a notebook at the ready, we set off to hear my fate.

My oncologist, new and hoping to make his mark in this big world of consultancy, was serious and matter-of-fact.

There was no small talk, no happy chatter. I knew straight away that what he would tell me was going to hurt. I was so glad I was armed with Erica and her notebook.

From what followed, I can remember only two things – I was to have six sessions of chemotherapy, carried out at three weekly intervals, and I would lose my hair.

With that information to contend with, there was no room for any more. For my own protection, I shut down.

I do remember asking if I could drink alcohol – who knows why I would ask that, but it seemed important at the time. The answer was 'Yes, do whatever you want to get yourself through this. Make sure you have some good times.' Because the rest is going to be awful, read between the lines …

I also asked if I could hold newborn babies when on chemotherapy. Two of my sisters-in-law were expecting imminently, and somehow it seemed a worthwhile question. Of course, the answer was yes.

What I didn't hear, Erica wrote down for me. She asked questions, noted answers, remained in the room while my mind wandered to a far nicer place where I could curl up in the sun and forget all this was happening.

'Is there anything you are particularly worried about?'

Em, yes … my hair … it's beautiful … is this really necessary? Menopause … what… I'm 40 .. surely not? No periods … really … well, I suppose that's a bonus!

There were other perks too, we decided … no haircuts … no shampoo or conditioner … the chance to try out some new hairstyles …. Perhaps I'd get two new looks and keep everyone guessing??

That afternoon seemed interminable and terrifying … with one redeeming feature. I met Val.

Val is my Breast Cancer Care nurse. As soon as I met her I knew she was the person I had been looking for to lead me through this minefield. I even liked her voice on the phone. She is kind, gentle, understanding, serious, bubbly, all the qualities you'd want from a nurse but very rarely find in one person.

I asked if she would take over my case, I wrote to request as much, and she joined my ranks of supporters, leading from the front in her own inimitable way – actually if I'm honest, I think I led from the front most of the time, but Val was always there at my shoulder, gently pushing me forward, providing someone to lean on if I fell back a little and taking the lead if I was struggling. She was the perfect ally through treatment, she is now my friend - and I am so grateful we found each other.

After that initial appointment with the oncologist, Val took Erica, her quickly filling notebook and I around the hospital. Trekking the endless corridors for chest x-rays, to pick up a voucher for an NHS wig (not as bad as it sounds thankfully – the memory I had of the dreaded National Health spectacles when I was ten didn't fill me with hope – a fear that was unfounded), and then up to the chemotherapy ward to meet up with the charge nurse, I entrusted myself to her kindness.

At that point, I needed someone to lean on … someone who had the knowledge and the wherewithal to pull me through this, and to give me the confidence to do it in my own way.

Val was that person …

**Hi Sonja. Just heard your news. I am so sorry. I can't put into words what I want to say but we are holding you close in our hearts and want you to know how much we are thinking of you. Anything at all that we can do, anytime at all, please please just shout. We are all here for you in any way that we can be. Take care. Love and very big hugs.**
**Rachel, sister-in-law X**

I left the hospital with Erica and went straight back into the throng of a children's birthday party.

By that time, Emma and Matthew knew I had a lump, and Emma whispered in the matter-of-fact way that only the innocence of being seven can bring: "I told everyone you were at the hospital to see about your lump, but I didn't tell them where it was. I didn't want you to be embarrassed."

Out of the mouths of babes…

**Sonja. Thinking of you. Will keep praying.**
**I know you can beat this.**
**Karen, friend X**

A few renditions of Happy Birthday to You later, the fairies left and a stillness descended on the house. I knew I had to tell the children something. They were expecting to hear how I'd got on at the hospital, so I told them as much as I knew.

"You know I have a lump? Well the doctor says he needs to shrink it. The way he's going to shrink it is by giving me very strong medicine. The medicine will kill the lump, okay?"

The next bit I said very quickly – as much to protect myself as for the children:

"The only thing is, the medicine will make my hair fall out. But you can come with me and choose a cool wig. That okay too? Will you help me?"

Emma, being a girl and being younger, was quite happy with this idea. She seemed excited at the whole prospect. I'd obviously done a good sales job.

Matthew on the other hand, was worried – about himself. "What will my friends say if you come to school with a bald head? They'll laugh at me."

Inside, I was crying. Why should my children have to go through this – why should I have to go through this? Why? Why?

Outside, the mummy in me took over. "Matthew, I wouldn't come to school with a bald head. I don't want people to laugh at me either. I promise I'll look the same – I'll look like me whatever happens. Okay? Deal?"

He was happier, and I vowed to myself then that whatever happened, I wouldn't let them down.

Val asked me recently if I thought I'd managed to keep that promise. 'Yes,' I answered. 'Sometimes I thought I wouldn't, but I really think I did."

"I think you did too," she agreed, and we got all teary together.

**Keep strong, be positive. You will get through this. Catriona, friend X**

# Emma Read

## My daughter was seven when my breast cancer was diagnosed. She told me her memories.

"I was trying not to be sad when mummy got breast cancer, but I was sad inside. I tried to forget about it and have a nice time.

I liked the books mummy and I read together, and we did lots of drawing too. We spent more time together than we usually do, because mummy didn't go out so much so we had plenty of time to do craft.

I thought her wigs were really nice – and now I wear them for dress up. I do think she looks nicer without her wig on because she's got very nice hair.

When mum first took her wig off and she had very short hair, my cousin Eliza said 'You look like a boy'. It was a bit of a shock for us all, especially people who hadn't seen her looking like that, but everyone got used to it.

I had seen her with a bald head, although she usually wore a hat because her head got cold. She looked alright like that but I'm glad none of my friends saw her like that because I think mum would have been embarrassed.

On my birthday, mum couldn't be there because she was at the hospital. I was turning seven and I had a fun time at my party, but I had a big shock afterwards when mum came home and told us that she had breast cancer. She got it on my birthday. I think I'll always remember that.

Dad did my party, and he did all the party games. He was really good at everything – we did some craft, and sucking up sweeties with straws. It was funny. Mummy planned it all, and daddy was in charge on the day.

My friends wondered where mum was, and I told them she was at the hospital but I didn't say why because I didn't want to have to tell them she had a lump in her breast. I thought she'd be embarrassed.

I took the book Mummy's Got A Lump, and another book called Mum has Breast Cancer, into school and my teacher read them to me while the rest of the class were at Assembly. It helped me to speak to my teacher about it because she listened and said things that made me happy. I didn't worry so much when I told my teacher. I knew my mum was going to get better because she told me that. I wasn't worried that she would die, I never even thought about it.

I didn't tell my friends because I didn't really want to. I was trying to forget about it so I didn't want to talk about it all the time to my friends. Someone in my class said their gran had died of breast cancer and that made me sad and worried. I thought it was better not to talk about the sad stories.

When we were out in the caravan with Auntie Erica, we sat and we had chips and chicken nuggets from the chip shop and had a chat. It was kind of like a bedtime story and it did help a lot to speak to someone who loves mummy just like we do.

The day that mummy left us at Auntie Erica's caravan to go for chemotherapy, she was crying lots. I was really sad that day, and really worried about what was going to happen to mummy. She gave me a special necklace to cheer me up.

When I thought about it in a good way, mummy was going to have a treat as well. She got the needle in her hand for an hour, but then she got a massage afterwards and she got to read some magazines with her friends.

Mum felt very sick after chemotherapy and stayed in bed sometimes, but that was okay too because we did drawing in bed and read books. I liked spending time with mum in the house, doing lots of fun activities.

I did lots of nice things – I went to my friends' houses for tea and for sleepovers, and I was still able to go to dancing and Beavers. Those things helped me forget about mummy being ill.

I also went to the Clan Children's Group, which gave the chance to do lots of nice things. We have been to the carnival, the beach, the cinema, the theatre, and lots of workshops. The Clan Children's Group helps children by cheering them up if they have someone at home who has cancer, or if someone they love has died of cancer. It helps you make lots of new friends and it does make you happy. I just wanted to be like everyone else.

I remember watching mummy at the Bling Fling and being really proud of her. We helped decorate her clothes for it with sequins and sparkles. On the day of the Bling Fling, we watched everybody warming up and walking onto the railway line, and then we got to stay in the park much later than usual.

Lots of mummy's friends took her out for nice dinners and bottles of wine and things when she had breast cancer. All her friends made her laugh.

If your mummy has breast cancer, I would say to look after her, and try to forget about it by playing nice games. I think we helped mummy by making her smile and doing nice things for her.

# Chapter 6

**You are very much in our thoughts. Like the sunflowers with their faces up to the sun, we hope the sun shines on you throughout the coming weeks – Card from my Uncle Bill and Auntie Rhoda**

The day after I learned my fate for the next few months, a sense of calm descended. I felt I was all cried out. I had chosen my funeral hymns and readings over the weeks' of waiting time, and now that had come to an end, suddenly a sense of control kicked in.

Being the kind of person who likes having plans, I was far happier. I had dates for the diary and targets to work towards. Although Val was advising me to 'Take every day as it comes', I am the kind of person who thrives on a timetabled existence. And at last, my period in limbo had come to an end. I was happier than I'd been in weeks...

So when my friend Pam asked if I was up to cycling out the old railway line, it felt like the best idea in the world. And of course, the promise of tea and cake at the end of our journey is always an incentive for a girl like me...

Four of us made that trip – Lesley, Pam, Lisa and I – who, along with another two friends Janine and Lorraine, ended up making up the Bling Fling committee. But that was way down the line. For the moment, we were friends, having fun, enjoying the sun and sharing laughs and chatter as if all the worry was behind us. Looking on, no one would have guessed the battle that lay ahead. But for the moment, we were living, and enjoying life – and that was the single, most important thing to all of us.

The day was sunny, and a local secondary school was out en masse on a sponsored walk, hundreds of teenagers having to move aside to let this merry band of laughing cyclists through.

At one point I met two teacher friends whom I have known for years. As I cycled past, roaring my greetings with a backward glance and a toss of the head, my long hair flew in the wind and I felt beautiful, happy and on top of the world.

I remember it crossed my mind at that moment that no one would see me like that again for years – perhaps ever. The reality of losing my hair loomed ominously, but for now, I could forget and put the past few weeks of worry behind me, setting myself up for the next 18 weeks - to chemotherapy and beyond.

**Dearest Sonja, We'll be thinking of you over the next 18 weeks. Keep positive – be strong, be bold, be beautiful – be You! Skerry, Michael, Elliot and Daniel X**

Janine is an old friend who has been a big part of my life for the last 20 years. She's one of those people that you don't remember meeting, it seems like she's always been there sharing a coffee, some words of wisdom, a laugh…

Although I don't remember exactly how we met, I do remember hitting it off with her instantly, and spending the next year going to weekly aerobics classes, and afterwards, cementing our friendship over chocolate fudge cake and diet drinks which made all that hard work worthwhile. Our shared love of food has always been our secret bond, I suspect, and dinner parties with Janine at the helm were a calendar highlight in those pre-children years.

Match-making is also a forte – a fact of which Graham and I are living proof. We met one Christmas at a Murder Mystery Party chez Janine – a date that was fully set up to maximise the chance of our meeting. At that time, it seemed every special occasion called for a group of relative strangers to dress up, get into character and solve a make-believe crime with friends they'd just met. Graham was Janine's neighbour in those heady days of tenement living, and seeing in him a nice guy and musician to boot – my talented husband plays the piano beautifully - she invited him along, then sat back and watched as our romance unfolded. Personally, I think she just wanted something interesting to twitch her curtains at, but she denies that is so - and I'll never know for sure, as in time she got what she wanted.

Graham was dressed as an actor, Cecil Bidet Mille, while I was Herbaceous Border the gardener, complete with tatty clothes, welly boots and stubble, painted on with gusto by my wee sister Heidi. Quite obvious why he was attracted to me ... I really did look my best that night. Well he must have seen through the rather hastily thrown together attire, as eight months later we were engaged, and another eight months on, we became Mr and Mrs Read in front of our family and friends.

Over the years, Janine and I have formed the firmest of bonds, as have our children, who were born a year apart, and our husbands who struggle to fit a word in edgeways when we get together.

The Easter before my breast cancer was diagnosed, our families shared the experience of a lifetime - a cruise from New York to Panama on board the Queen Mary 2. This was a treat planned to celebrate my 40$^{th}$ birthday - and since Janine's wonderful mum lost her long battle with breast cancer seven years earlier, just before her 40$^{th}$ - we shared my special day instead.

Our combined families enjoyed two weeks in the lap of Cunard luxury, wining, dining and dressing to impress in ballgowns and jewel-encrusted necklaces - costume jewellery of course, but with enough sparkle to earn me the title Mrs Bling among the friends who are close enough to be allowed to tease me whatever I'm going through...

As well as the name, which would stick and inspire my whole persona over the coming year, that holiday also gave me memories into which I could escape during some of the worst moments of treatment. Whenever my emotional state would spiral out of control, or my fears grew too much to handle, I found myself in the piano bar of my mind, sipping cocktails while the world slipped by under a Caribbean sunset.

When I was first diagnosed, Janine took on the positive role I always knew she would, and gave me the benefit of her experience of help available to cancer sufferers in Aberdeen - she took me to CLAN (Cancer Link Aberdeen and North), a haven in the centre of our northern city which welcomes anyone affected by cancer.

We didn't make a big deal of it I seem to remember - we dropped in while we were passing CLAN House on the way to a shopping mall – doing a bit of retail therapy, which always helps when a girl is feeling less than her sparkling best.

Stepping inside Clan House is, as it says on the tin, like stepping into a haven. A haven from the medical world, from being a mum, from being a wife and from the hustle and bustle of everyday life which continues even when you are going through cancer treatment. It was the one place, apart from the hospital, where I felt I had the opportunity to come to terms with what I was going through, to speak to others who understood and weren't hurt or offended by what I had to say, and where I could find the emotional support to help me deal with the physical treatment I was going through.

From my first mug of peppermint tea within the peaceful confines of the converted church in which CLAN is housed, I felt at home there. The gentle sound of an indoor waterfall, the hypnotic sight of a giant fish tank bubbling with fresh water and constantly moving with life, and the kindly band of volunteers always on hand with a cup of tea and a listening ear meant it quickly became my second home over the next few months.

And as well as time to chat, there were the therapies that CLAN offered – at this stage, when just starting out on chemotherapy, I was booked up for sessions with the Reflexologist and Aromatherapist, both new experiences and a perfect treat within my life which at the time seemed to be otherwise dictated by hospital appointments and bracing walks.

Reflexology was a surprising godsend – I say surprising because I have the tickliest feet in the history of tickly feet. When I was having my first baby, I remember failing miserably the Ante Natal Class challenge of preparing for childbirth by practising deep breathing while Graham tickled my toes. Every time, without fail, I ended up rolling around the floor with tears of laughter streaming down my face… Given the fact that Matthew was eventually born by Caesarean Section, you can see that my attempts during the actual birth were just as futile.

However, lying back while the reflexologist massaged my feet, describing her findings and clearing blockages throughout my body while touching pressure points first discovered by Egyptian doctors in biblical times, I felt so relaxed that occasionally, I have to admit, I fell asleep.

Even straight after chemotherapy, when I had a real problem with my bowels – sorry if you're reading this over a cup of tea and a light snack, but chemo is not just about presents and magazine reading as

I'm sure you'll appreciate – reflexology came to the rescue. I'd tried the natural laxatives and even the chemical ones (not something I've ever done before, but did end up resorting to in my attempt not to try to become a superhero), with precious little result, until finally the reflexologist came to my rescue. How she managed to shift my load (told you it wasn't pleasant) by massaging my feet, I'll never know, but take it from me, half an hour later I felt great inside – and had perfectly soft feet to show for it. Result.

And then there was Aromatherapy, in which a masseur uses essential oils to massage the head, back, hands and arms, and each time I felt like a new woman. Pampered, preened and all the things you feel after a trip to a good hairdresser. In fact, given my lack of hair at the time, I suppose my trips to CLAN House were my only chance of enjoying that kind of attention that every woman wants and needs in her life. The physical closeness seemed to open up conversations too – and in the way that many clients reveal precious secrets to their hairdressers, so too the therapists at CLAN become entrusted with the fears and worries of their clients going through cancer treatment. To prepare them for this responsibility, everyone who works or volunteers at CLAN is trained in counselling skills, and the non-threatening, laid back atmosphere makes it the perfect place to think, talk and take time to digest and ponder what is going on around you.

As far as I was concerned, CLAN House provided an escape from hospital appointments and the rest of my life, in which I was often still trying to be everything for everyone – as much as you try to calm down and take it easy, being a wife, mother, family member and friend doesn't stop when you've got cancer. And nor do you want to it to... for those are exactly the things that make the treatment endurable.

## Carol's Story

**Carol has been an aromatherapist at Clan House for four years. She explained her role in the cancer journey**

When people come to Clan House, they are looking for something to help them get through the whole trauma of cancer and the medical treatments involved. As therapists, we are not actually treating the cancer itself – we leave that to the medical professionals. What we do is treat the whole person and the physical and emotional challenges that come with having cancer.

There are many physical challenges that our clients may be going through during and after medical treatments, such as radiotherapy, chemotherapy and surgery. Some of these challenges include extreme fatigue, nausea, pains, constipation, diarrhoea, sensitive and/or fragile skin, hair loss, peripheral neuropathy (tingling, numbness and a sensation of 'pins and needles' in the hands and feet), lymphodema, scars and adhesions.

They may also have central lines, catheters and stomas fitted. Our massage treatments are tailored to take into account all of the above and, where we can, help to alleviate some of the side effects of their medical treatments.

When clients come for therapy at Clan, they are seen in a private room - there's soft music, soft towels and they have the space and time to do what they want to do. If they want to cry, they can do that. If they want to talk or vent anger, they can do that too. If they want to do neither, if they just want to enjoy the therapy then it's their time and they can do what they want with it.

As therapists, we give people freedom to be themselves. Some people come to see me, and they are just in the room for a few seconds when everything comes out. That happens for various reasons. Some have nobody else to talk to, others have plenty of people to talk to but they feel that nobody is listening or understanding what they are saying.

Others enjoy the actual therapy itself, but they don't open up emotionally for a long time. They'll speak about anything else except the cancer because that's what they want and need to do. Everyone eventually needs to speak about what they're going through – it may take two years (and it has done in some cases) – but people always need to let their feelings out at some point in their life.

My work at CLAN is totally different from my work with private clients – people who are dealing with cancer have all faced death, and there's no pretence – there's a real honesty about what they've been through. Yes, they want to talk about minor things as well, because that's their way of coping, but they speak openly and from the heart.

The strength and courage of the people I've met through CLAN is awesome. People who are being treated for cancer are going through something massive, their whole life is changing, everything is changing – their perception, their relationships with everybody around them. Sometimes that happens on a subtle level, sometimes it's like a bus hitting them.

There are some who will take it on the chin and move on as and when they are ready, but others will move backwards and forwards as they go. As therapists, our role is quite simple. We support people through their journey - we don't guide or advise, we just support. You can see 'Aha' moments as they are talking. You watch as they suddenly realise something that makes sense to them – either 'I can do this' or 'That's not what I want' – and as they talk, they work it out for themselves.

The journey continues long after treatment. Dealing with cancer changes people, mostly for the better – almost 100% for the better. The people we see in CLAN House are the ones who have accepted they have cancer and take control of it. We help them for that time and eventually there comes a time when they pull back from us because they no longer need us in the same way.

If someone is dying of cancer, there is still a journey and the time we spend with them is even more precious. I have been privileged over the last four years to speak with people about the dying process, and that is something very special indeed. People who open up to us have come to terms with the fact that they are dying. There are some who just don't want to talk about it. You also see the ones who have switched off and are just coming in because they're doing it for others, for their family, to keep them happy.

As therapists, we also treat carers of people dying of cancer, which is slightly different again. In that case, the therapies don't have to be tailored because they're not having medical treatment, but the emotional impact is sometimes worse than on the person who has cancer – they're dealing with it on a different level. This is especially the case in someone who has cared to the death point of their loved one, because their last living memory of that person is their last breath, and it takes them a long time to move past that point. They're not getting the attention or the support, so it's a harder journey in a very different way. And it takes a long time – often years – for them to come to terms with that.

People come to CLAN House at their most vulnerable time – they've lost their hair, they've had massive confidence shattering surgery, or they've lost someone very close to them. The minute they come in for a therapy and take their clothes off for a massage, they feel exposed, and that leads to some very deep-rooted feelings and emotions rising to the surface... If I'm working on mastectomy scar tissue, people get very emotional about it. Often I'm the first person who has been allowed to touch their scar, and that is very moving.

For patients, it's nice to know that somebody accepts how you are, and they're not afraid to touch you. I will massage a scalp when someone takes off their wig – and all of them have done so far. That can be an emotional time as well.

It really is a privilege what we do here. There are people who come to Clan who have got nobody – either physically nobody, or people round them who think once the treatment's done they're okay - 'That's it, you should be back to normal'. But life is never normal again for anyone who has been through cancer – and really it's never normal for the carers either, even though they might not admit it. Cancer changes your outlook, everything shifts. You have to build new boundaries round your relationships. Sometimes people don't have the strength to do that within themselves – but coming here gives them the strength to deal with their life.

When I first met Sonja, she had just finished chemotherapy, and had stopped wearing her wig. I think she was always a confident person, but I feel that now, months down the line, there is a new confidence in her, having been through her own breast cancer journey. She's grown, she's changed a little, she's opened up in some ways and let some people closer... and she's more precious about where she goes, what she does and who she spends her time with.

That's nice to see because you can see contentment in her, a settlement. I feel she's opened up space in her life for her now, rather than being a mum, being a friend, being a family member and relative. There's now a bit of Sonja in there too, and time for her. There's great strength there, but there's also contentment, and that's so important...

## Chapter 7

**How does it feel to be radioactive? Hot stuff! Heidi**

Strangely, naively perhaps, it hadn't dawned on me yet that the lump may not be the only sign of cancer in my body.

When the oncologist booked me in for a full body scan on all my major organs, and a radioactive tracer to check my heart, I thought he was getting baseline assessments from which to start my chemotherapy course. Seems not...

I arrived, having just had a plate of soup with mum, to discover I was supposed to be there with an empty stomach. Typical. Never have been much good at reading instructions ...

However, 'because I was nice and slim' - the radiographer's words, not mine, although they work well with me I can assure you! - the scan could still take place. Liver ... check .... Stomach .... check ... ovaries and womb ... check ... anything else he could find to scan ... check. All present and correct, and looking absolutely healthy ... fit even.

Somewhere along the way, I realised what they were looking for but thankfully hadn't found, and wondered how, just how, could I have one tiny lump of cancer. Where had it come from? Why on earth did my cells choose to begin behaving badly in that particular place, when the rest of my body was happily healthy?

Although it doesn't make sense - even now that I've had months to reflect on it all - I am of course grateful that the cancer cells elsewhere in my body kept themselves under control. It's just the breast ones that forgot ...

The radioactive tracer turned out to be a couple of needles in my arm – I was beginning to feel like a pin cushion, but nothing compared to what was to come over the next few months - followed by a trip through a huge scanning machine.

I lay there for five minutes, wired for sound, while a tracer checked my heart rate and classical music calmed me, lulling me into a mode of deep relaxation – the first time I'd rested for a couple of weeks.

I emerged to the not unexpected news that my heart was healthy, I was obviously very fit and – again – it must be quite a shock.

What? A shock for them too? Where did those blueberries go wrong?

**Hope it went okay today. If you fancy a manicure on me later if docs think it's okay, just call X Lesley**

I was radioactive for 24 hours after the heart scan, and so told not to have prolonged close contact with the children - as in not to cuddle them for hours on end, something I had not done since their toddler days but had done a lot more of since my diagnosis. For their sake and mine, Erica took them to Dingwall in the North of Scotland for a holiday weekend, giving them some fun time away from the week's anxieties, and removing any chance of my using them as a personal comfort blanket.

Lesley, who had been planning her daughter's Pink and Pearly nails party, invited me along to enjoy a manicure, very sweetly (as is her nature) making up for the fact that I had missed Emma's birthday celebration a few days before.

Anyone who knows me, would know that even a radioactive blast couldn't keep me away from a free manicure – and knowing that I wouldn't be tempted, or indeed get the chance to cuddle any of the excited eight-year-old party-goers that afternoon – I joined the happy throng of merrymakers to get myself blinged up for my first chemotherapy session.

Bright pink nails have always had their own form of healing for a girl like me ... and I came out of that manicure feeling a million dollars. Just what every girl needs when starting out on the fight of her life...

Thinking about you all the time. You're being very brave although I realise you don't have much choice. Manicure sounds good. Lots of love Fiona X


PS Stephen says to send you lots of love. He was very upset by your news and is amazed by how you're coping so far. You're fab. X Fiona

## Chapter 8

### Mummy's got a lump...

So says the book for children, which is standard issue for any mum going through the treatment of breast cancer. Produced by the NHS, it gives an account of the story, in child-friendly terms, but using all the words they would come across along the way.

The way I handled the issue of breast cancer with my children was very much led by this book. After the first night, strong medicine became chemotherapy, and then chemo, as we all got more familiar with the three-weekly routine.

Eventually, it was tripping off their tongues – 'Mum's getting chemo today … she's feeling a bit sick … she's tired … yes, dad's taking us because mum's a bit tired today … poor mum has a really sore mouth, but her good week is coming up.'

To begin with, I knew the children would need help to cope with the news of my breast cancer, and as they spend more than half their day at school, I realised some of their questions were sure to emerge there.

One of my first tasks, as I saw it, was to tell the school, and more specifically the children's teachers.

Matthew was mad at me – 'Why do you have to tell everybody? It's so embarrassing.' It's the talk of breasts that gets him every time – typical boy!

But Emma went off to class that morning armed with the aforementioned book, and had a quiet moment in the reading corner, while the rest of the class were at assembly, discussing her worries.

Matthew, for all his embarrassment, took the lead from his little sister. He went and collected the book when Emma was finished with it, and read it with his young and very beautiful teacher who helped him find out the facts about breast cancer from the computer.

This turned out to be the perfect pitch with Matthew – why didn't I think of it? When he discovered from Google that most people are cured of the disease – in fact, current statistics say that only 15% of those diagnosed with breast cancer will die of it (still too many but it is improving all the time, thanks to research) – and his teacher assured him that I was young and fit and perfectly placed to get through it, he was a changed boy. He suddenly believed and was on side again ... and thankfully, that's where he stayed throughout the journey.

**All fine so far ... just cycled to Tesco – five bikes in a row. Felt like Von Trapps! Text from Erica in Dingwall X**

Yes, the children were having fun in Dingwall, and, sporting the pinkest nails any caravan site anywhere has ever seen, I spent a night with them there the weekend before chemotherapy began.

I arrived after a lovely drive with Erica's brother and sister-in-law, Kenny and Maggie – a drive that was often punctuated with coffee shop trips along the way. The weather was beautiful and we were in no rush ... life slows down when you've had a traumatic few weeks.

For the first half hour after we arrived, my niece Eliza looked thoughtfully at me, in the intense, probing way that she has got down to a fine art. At five, she is the sandwich child – a girl fighting for her place between two boisterous brothers – and I have always had a special place in my heart for her.

As her godmother, I feel I have done my duty well, and I love the way she questions everything, takes all news in, processes it carefully and then drip feeds it into conversations, enticing us to discuss at great length – because she needs to.

It dawned on me instantly that the book Emma had declared as her new favourite read – Mummy Has A Lump – had become a lifeline for the pair of them that weekend, and together they had discussed, digested and, in Eliza's case, memorised all the important bits (in her eyes anyway).

So when she said 'It's not your fault you've got breast cancer, Auntie Sonja – you didn't catch it from anyone you know…" I knew she had read and understood the book and was now using it to counsel me.

And then there was the drawing of the mummy in the book, sitting with a bald head, her wig flung casually over the bedpost… a thrill for the girls by this time, who were anticipating with slightly morbid curiosity the bald-headed me that was yet to come …

**Had a lovely weekend in Dingwall – just what the doctor (and patient) ordered … weather was fab. Sonja XX**

The Moray Firth shimmered in the sunshine as we walked, talked and had fun together, collected Autumn leaves and berries, spotting dolphins – all the while gathering stunning memories to see me through the worst of the days ahead.

And it was while we were there that the robin first came …

I say first because I have been visited by a robin at many stages over the last few months, always when I've been particularly down, or have heard some good news. Strangely, the first time it happened was the day before chemotherapy.

We were sitting in the caravan's awning eating breakfast. The weather was bright, sunny even – something of an Indian summer late in September.

As we sat chatting, a robin hopped in beside the table and looked around. We went silent, wondering at its bravery, watching for all of 30 seconds as it sat still, looking at me, cocked its head cheekily and then hopped off.

I looked at Erica and, through tears, breathed; 'Everything's going to be alright. You know that, don't you?'

**Hey Erica, Thanks for having kids – and me – this weekend. Love you, Sonja X**

# Children's Counsellors, CLAN

**Eileen and Leigh work together at CLAN House to provide a support for children who are affected by cancer. Aberdeen is unique in that it has specialist support for young people, and the women are in great demand helping them cope with the effect cancer has on lives and families. They told me about the rewarding work they do.**

"Children all react to a cancer diagnosis differently. Some children are very matter-of-fact about everything and if you give them the facts, they're happy and off they go with that knowledge and deal with it. Others take some time to absorb it and start asking questions. Others will ask all the questions and then say 'Okay, can I go and ride my bike now?' and you're left thinking 'Did they not understand what I said?' Well yes, they did but they're dipping in and out of what's going on and sticking with their normal routine which gives them security.

"Sometimes when children ask questions, adults assume they have to give them a long explanation or explain the whole process. In actual fact, if children have only one question and you answer that one question, they're not interested in hearing anything else so they go off because they've got what they wanted out of the conversation. Sometimes adults aren't particularly good at hearing what children want to know. They assume – maybe because they've rehearsed it in their head or they want them to know what they think is important – that they should tell them everything. Telling children can go very differently from how people think it will go."

I wondered if it was important that the person who has cancer should take responsibility for telling the children, as I did – or if it matters if that task falls to someone else.

"It depends on how well the person with cancer is able to answer the questions. If the person who has cancer is distressed and upset that is not very good for the children. I'm not saying that they should never see you cry or get upset, but if you're able to keep it simple and keep a check on your emotions, it's usually better for the parents to tell the children themselves."

Now that the whole cancer journey has ended, my daughter Emma has taken to wearing my wig. Seeing her with my long red locks makes me feel a little uncomfortable – brings back memories of a time I'd rather forget. But Leigh believes my daughter's fascination with my wig is a positive thing. "It's definitely a positive thing because it means she has no unhappy memories relating to that time when you were wearing your wig. Maybe at the same time, she also feels close to you in a way by wearing the wig. She wants to feel what you experienced so she can relate to it."

Both of the children have had great fun at the CLAN Children's Group, which organises events and activities for children affected by cancer. Eileen remembers how the group came about.

"The reason it started – or one of the reasons anyway – is because it can be quite isolating when an adult, or someone the children knows, has cancer. The group was formed to give children time to mix with other children, not having to explain anything – they don't have to talk because the focus is social and having fun, nothing is asked of them at all and they can just be themselves."

Although the group is not designed for heavy chat, it can just happen, says Eileen. "Sometimes children talk to one another and real friendships develop there. Some are still in touch long after they stop coming to CLAN."

Children often struggle to talk with anyone else about cancer, says Eileen: "Children have really good, close friends but cancer is not something they want to talk about normally with their friends. Teenagers might tell one or two close friends.

"Adults have their own way of dealing with things, and their own outlets. The Clan Children's Group is an outlet for children - in fact, this might be the only outlet for some children being affected by cancer. They might come from a low income family who couldn't partake in these activities normally because they couldn't afford to. Often there's less income because a parent is going through cancer treatment. Maybe their life is spent between going to school and going to the hospital, so the Children's Group gives them the chance to spend two hours being children, acting their age, playing with other children.

"A lot of children grow up very quickly when their parents get cancer because they're in a very adult environment, hearing very adult conversations with medical words they've never heard of. It's nice for them to have fun and to feel able and relaxed enough to have fun without feeling guilty."

When speaking to my own children about cancer treatment, I made sure I used all the terminology as it was said to me. Eileen, who wrote one of the books I used with my children, believes this is by far the best approach: "If people use different euphemisms it's confusing. Using the appropriate word is always the best thing. You can simplify it to begin with, as Sonja did, like using the words 'strong medicine' and then move onto chemotherapy, and chemo as it becomes less scary and more familiar.

"The words are big words and they sound quite scary – they sound like a big thing and they are a big thing, but children don't know what the big thing is. It could mean anything to a child. It's adults that have the problem. Some adults believe you can't say the c-word to children: "It's a secret they shouldn't know about". Children always know when something is wrong and sometimes if you don't tell them, they use their imagination and come up with something worse."

Eileen believes children often deal better than adults with cancer treatment. "Children are so at ease with it, which can catch you out because you don't want them to be so familiar with such things when they are so young. But it's just part of what's going on and they're just adding to their experience of life."

"Parents sometimes ask us to get involved and actually their children are doing fine. Sometimes we find they're not talking to their parents about it at all. Instead they're talking to a friend, a teacher, someone else they're close to. They're not in denial with what's going on and they are dealing with it, but in a way that's right for them."

Classically, the problems can come after treatment ends, says Eileen. "It can have repercussions later on – just as it can for everyone. Children know if you're going to the hospital, the doctors are keeping an eye on you, they're checking up on you. When it all ends, there can be that fear sets in because you're not being checked. Sometimes they're not consciously thinking these things but it's all going on in their head."

As with everything else to do with cancer, the way your family deals with it will be personal and unique to your own situation.

Says Leigh: "The best way to get through cancer is the best way for you as a family. What might be right for some may be totally wrong for somebody else, but the important thing is to do what is right for your family at the time."

# Chapter 9

**Hi Sonj. All the best for tomorrow. We are all thinking about you. Gav X**

**Thanks Gav, Crapping myself to be honest but I'll be brave. Sonja X**

I break out in a cold sweat even thinking about the night before chemotherapy started.

I don't know what I expected, to be honest ... an instant attack of hair fallout? Three weeks spent crouched over a toilet, only to begin again with the next dose? The end of life as we know it?

Whatever it was never materialised thankfully, but it didn't stop me crying myself to sleep that night, and then waking every hour until the dawn.

As I lay, clockwatching, desperate for that interminable night to end, I came to a decision which shaped my whole approach to chemotherapy over the next few months.

I decided there was only one way for me to do this – in style.

As the sun rose, I got to work. Dressing to impress in colour from head to toe - red shoes, pink nail varnish and the brightest necklace I could find on my groaning jewellery stand.

My make-up was applied with as much care as on my wedding day, and I curled my beautiful long hair as if I was hitting the town on a Saturday night.

Finally I was ready to take the chemotherapy ward by storm.

**Went to sleep thinking about you and woke up thinking about you. Hope you get through today okay. The battle begins! Lots and lots of love, Fiona X**

**Good luck this afternoon. You are the best! Lesley**

**Thinking about you. Kids send all their love. Erica X**

Every three weeks brought a new chemo buddy – a friend carefully chosen to make me smile while the chemo nurses were dosing me up with the hard stuff.

The first was Nicola, my self-professed 'ginger witch', who knew almost as soon as I did that I had breast cancer, and who always believed – and told me often – that I would get through it.

Nicola is a stunning redhead with a beautiful personality to match. She is full of fun and chatter, and says all the things that are guaranteed to make a girl feel good.

A few weeks before I was diagnosed with breast cancer, Nicola's husband secured a job overseas, and although she was orchestrating the family's move to Kuala Lumpur – a not altogether small task, given her three children, two cats, house to rent out and new abode to find - she wouldn't have me go to my first session without her.

How glad I was she insisted ... that first chemotherapy session set the standard of day out I came to expect over the next few months.

**Good luck for today babe. I'm expecting you to be fully up to date with the celebrity gossip after all the mag reading. Skerry X**

Nicola picked me up, like me, dressed to impress and armed with celebrity magazines, chocolate, drinks, strawberries and the first of my many chemotherapy presents – a beautiful corsage bracelet, specially chosen for me at Notting Hill market during a recent weekend in London.

Of course, I wore it – stylish to the end - and groomed to perfection for our big day, we entered the chemo ward as if we were celebrity guests at an Oscar Night party. I don't think the staff had any idea what had hit them ...

**Hope you do not feel instantly poisoned today. Thinking of you. Heidi X**

Well my darling sister, I didn't feel instantly poisoned... bit of an anti-climax after all that worry, actually.

The drugs were administered through a canula in my hand by a lovely young nurse who seemed to enjoy our chat over the celebrity magazines – concentrating all the time of course. We didn't let her join in too much – one must be sensible in such situations!

As she injected, she told me what they would do – 'This is the one which gives you a nasty taste in your mouth,' 'This one makes your hair fall out', 'Both kill all the fast-growing cells in your body – cancer, white blood cells, hair follicles, you name it. If it moves fast, it's a goner'. Well I added that last bit, but that's the result I was hoping for ...

One made my nose run, one gave me an instantly metallic taste, one made my bottom tingle – don't ask – but none were unbearable or gruelling in the least.

We left the ward just as we had entered - glamorous, smiling and happy - with the overriding feeling that we'd shared something special. A girls' day out that we'd never forget...

**To all my friends...**

**Just finished first chemotherapy... Feel absolutely fine. Long may it continue! Sonja X**

**Way to go girl! Skerry**

## Nicola's Story

The morning Sonja first came round to tell me her news, I distinctly remember the overpowering smell of fresh paint ... you see, we were getting organised to move to Kuala Lumpur and after a few fleeting weeks, our house was finally looking like the showhome I had always longed for – sadly not for us to enjoy but for the new tenants who'd move in in our wake...

Outside, it was one of those beautiful, fresh and crisp mornings in the Granite City, made complete with the sight of Sonja coming through our front gate, looking as gorgeous and radiant as ever – glowing as she does, from the inside out.

"Great," I thought. "I'll just put the kettle on ... a coffee with an old friend would be just the thing this morning." Something seemed to stop then - like a movie picture in slow motion, as I heard the ominous words - 'I've got breast cancer.' Truth be told, my first thought was undeniably "Oh Shit!"

Sonja calmly told me how she wasn't sure when to tell me as she didn't want to spoil the excitement of my move to KL. Spoiling anything was the last thing on my mind – I was glad to be given the chance to do my bit for her before I left.

I asked if I could go along to the first chemo session. Crikey! Chemo? We have all heard the word, approached it as 'something that happens to someone else', but this was the first time it was here, on my doorstep. Someone I knew well, had planned birthday parties for and shared the joys and horrors of parenting with was about to enter into that drug ridden world – and I had to help her to deal with it, whatever 'it' was.

The following week, it all began. The September holiday Monday was sunny for once and I packed Belgian chocolates, trashy celeb magazines and organic fruit drinks - normally it would be some alcoholic fizz for a girls' day out, but I wasn't sure if this would be allowed. I had picked up a wee bracelet for Sonja too for the occasion.

I wanted to make the appointment as fun and light-hearted as possible – that seemed important somehow, to do something we both enjoyed to get through an afternoon that I knew would probably be the least enjoyable thing we'd ever done together.

As we entered the chemo ward, it struck me how much younger Sonja was than everyone else, which got me thinking, this is so unfair. Why her? Why this age? We'd only just celebrated her 40th birthday, I had the remnants of that girls' shopping day in Edinburgh still rumbling around in the bottom of my handbag. This didn't make sense.

We were directed to a chair (which reminded me of those found in old people's homes) where it was all to happen. There, we met Sonja's assigned nurse – or poison giver of the day, who gave us the Cold Cap talk. She talked us through the options – would it save Sonja's hair, was it worth trying it? If she could put up with extreme cold as well as drugs coursing through her veins, would it make her fight a little easier? I remember wondering at the time 'What would I do?'

Sonja decided against it and we laughed about all the different new hairstyles she could wear. It was fun, but at the time I'm sure Sonja didn't really know how losing her hair would affect her – would anyone? When I broke my ankle some months later and I was complaining via Facebook about not being able to shave my legs, Sonja quickly and wittily replied 'At least you've got something to shave'! It certainly pays to count your blessings…

And then, the main event – what we had really come to see. The drugs. My abiding memory of that afternoon - and to this day I don't know why - was a plastic basin containing huge syringes filled with the poison, all looking toxic enough to wipe out a small community. Gosh there were so many, all emblazoned with names that sounded like toxic nuclear waste. Absolutely terrifying, but of course, I said none of that to Sonja.

Instead, as the nurse injected, we chatted and giggled our way through the first session, leaving all those goodies I had brought along untouched. Somehow eating and drinking was the last thing on either of our minds as we exchanged gossip and dreamed up future holidays in my soon-to-be new home.

Goodness knows what everyone thought of this giggling pair dressed to impress in the corner, but strange as it sounds we had a lovely afternoon together, time passed so quickly and the next thing we were driving back home.

I think I imagined the chemo drugs would have immediate effect – I might have to help Sonja to the car, stop to tend to her on the way home, at least have something that I'd have to deal with and reassure her about.

But amazingly, Sonja declared she felt no different… and we laughed as she received text after text from people happy to hear she had survived her first encounter with the chemo ward and perhaps more surprisingly, was still smiling…

A few weeks later, when I finally left Aberdeen for our new life, Sonja was still smiling and looking exactly the same – although, just as predicted, she lost her hair soon after I'd gone. Thankfully, although her hair went, she never did lose that positive approach to life that I knew would pull her through.

## Nicola's Resolutions at the end of the Year That Was:

Things I have learnt in 2009 or have been reminded about this year –
- Health is not to be taken for granted - look after that body of yours as you only get one
- Learn to live with disappointment and to move on
- Always say yes to sharing a cup of coffee with a friend - no matter how many things you had planned to do that day. You never know how much they might need you
- Respect all women

# Chapter 10

**Had a crap night sleep. Hope it was not a case of sibling ESP! Much love, Heidi X**
**Me too. Felt sick at 3 until I took an anti-sickness pill. Must be rattling by now! Fine this morning though. Kids coming with me to choose wig later. Lots of love Sonja X**

I did sleep relatively well the night after chemotherapy – catching up on the sleepless nights before, I guess. Once I knew I could handle it, I settled down to the task in hand, had an early night and swallowed all the anti-sickness pills I was allowed.

I decided early on in this adventure that I would follow Heidi's advice and go for the drugs. Take everything I was given, she advised, and I should get through this ordeal with my life and smile intact.

Now that the poison was in there, coursing around my body and looking for cells to attack, I knew I had to do something about my hair.

Some choose to wear what is called a 'cold cap', worn before, during and after chemotherapy to lower the temperature, stopping blood flowing so quickly to the hair follicles and in some absurd way, limiting hair loss.

I mulled this over and decided that because it would be impossible to look glam with a cold cap in situ, and more importantly because I hate being cold, I would go for the wig option instead.

This proved to be a good decision. I had minimum time to spend at the hospital, I always felt and looked normal when undergoing chemotherapy – and, perhaps best of all, I was able to reinvent myself three times over the next six months.

The first 'new me' was a glamorous redhead …

> **How are you and how did you get on at the wig fitting today? Nic X**

> **Fab Nicola. Thinking about going red in your absence. Going to do this in style!... Sonja**

> **Sonja, I would be very honoured if you went for red. Nic X**

The children and my friend Julie came with me to choose my new look on the day after chemotherapy.

Julie is a friend from my first ante-natal class. There are five of us – myself, Julie, Karen, Caroline and Catriona – who bonded over another of the toughest times in our life, becoming first-time mums.

The thoughts we didn't share at that time weren't worth speaking about. We knew everything about each other, shared laughs, compared notes and discussed in great detail the birth and nappy contents of our darling first-born child.

Nowadays the offspring themselves have grown up and grown apart, paths crossing occasionally on the football pitch or at cub camp, but not often enough to be considered close friends.

Not so for the mums, however. The chat has changed over the last ten years, but intrinsically we are the same – still helping each other out, now comparing marriages, parenting challenges, and embracing times of delight and despair with equal measure.

Julie's two boys were born three weeks after mine each time – some may say we planned it that way, but neither of us has ever been that organised.

Julie was the first of the group that I told about my breast cancer. I told her in the car on the way into town where we were meeting the others for lunch – not a particularly good move, but thankfully she had the wherewithal to park first before giving me a big hug.

Of course, like most, she was shocked and confused, but practicality being Julie's forte, she wanted to help. So she did - she chose my wig!

**Red hair! Sounds funky! Won't recognise you! Eva**

**Sounds fab, you'll be very foxy as a redhead! Rachel X**

The children had asked that I go for long hair. They wanted me to look the same, and at that time, that's what I wanted too.

Trying on wigs with my own hair underneath was not the easiest task I've ever undertaken. My own hair is thick and luscious (and long at the time, as I think I might have mentioned?) and stuffing it inside a tight wig reminded me of wearing a swimming cap to lessons as a child.

I tried long blonde Dolly (yes, the wigs have names) but somehow it didn't look like me. That girl in the mirror, strained, worried, too blonde for her own skin… it just didn't feel right. Strange as it was exactly the same colour as my hair at the time. And so I tried red Louise … Bingo! The perfect colour for the moment … and a redhead was born.

**Sonja, you're always stylish so no surprises there! Fiona X**

**Sounds fabulous darling! Skerry X**

**Hey Sonj. Long and red sounds fab. Be a change from natural blonde! Gav**

Ailsa is my neighbour across the road. She is a nurse and midwife, and has always been around to give sensible and down-to-earth advice on medical issues. She knows exactly what to say and how to help, without ever having to be asked, and so when she asked me over for a cup of tea and chat about the wig choosing, I took Louise with me for the ride.

It was a little weird –surreal even - showing Louise off before my own hair had actually fallen out. I'm not sure I even believed my hair would go at that stage … I certainly didn't feel the drugs at work. But they asked, and as I've never been one to shy away from an audience, I was happy to oblige. It was a boost when later I received this message from Ailsa, on behalf of her 12-year-old daughter.

**As I was saying goodnight to Rhona tonight she called me back. 'Actually mum, I think Sonja's hair is really cool' We hadn't been chatting about it at all – it was a totally spontaneous remark. Just thought you'd like to hear it too! Ailsa X**

**Thanks! I know kids are brutally honest so that means a lot. I'll wear it with pride! Sonja**

## Julie's Story

**Julie came along to my first wig fitting, armed with sweets and chatter. She looked after the children and gave me her verdict on my choices. Here is the day as she remembers it:**

When Sonja mentioned she was going for a wig fitting, I immediately offered to accompany her and help her choose something suitable. Her children would be coming too so I was determined it would be a fun outing despite the circumstances.

The 'salon' was hidden away inside an ordinary house in the centre of town, which had had the downstairs converted into a reception area and fitting rooms. I arrived first, feeling a bit apprehensive, which made we wonder how Sonja would be feeling.

When they arrived, the wig specialist Rose took Sonja through for an initial consultation while I chatted with Matthew and Emma. It became obvious that their main concern was that their mum would still look like their mum. I assured them she would look just as fabulous. Then we got the call to join Sonja in the consultation room...

What probably made it a bit easier for Sonja was that her hair hadn't started falling out. Perhaps if she'd had a bald head, she would have been less comfortable about us seeing her? As it was, it was a bit like going to the hairdresser for a new look. The lady brought out several wigs of varying colours and lengths and Sonja started trying them out. I can honestly say that there was not one that didn't suit her - there were some that looked better than others but all would have been acceptable.

There was a fabulous red bob which unfortunately Matthew was not so keen on but was my personal favourite and a gorgeous long blondish one that just screamed "celebrity"! It was all too enticing for Emma and I - we dived in and started trying on. However, the fitter's cries of how much they cost reeled us back in. Some were made from "real" hair (do people donate hair??) and got static when you brushed them.

Finally Sonja settled on one not dissimilar to her own hair which pleased the children and I think pleased Sonja (or was there a hankering for that racy red? Apparently there was, and she decided to go red, ordering Louise the wig in an auburn colour to give her a warm look for Autumn which would leave her glowing while the rest of us looked pale and washed out as winter set in).

We started discussing the benefits of a wig - no more bad hair days, looking dishevelled in the rain and wind, washing and drying every day to name but a few.

On the way out I treated her to some special shampoo and conditioner to keep it in tip-top condition and give her the excuse of 'staying in to wash her hair' if she needed it!"

I'm so glad Sonja chose the look she did – she looked fabulous throughout her treatment, giving her confidence and leaving her glowing no matter what she was going through. More than could be said for the rest of us... there were times we even envied that freshly washed at all times look...!

# Chapter 11

**How r u doing doll? Skerry**
**Still okay thanks, but really tired. Going to**
**bed soon. Running out of vases for all the**
**flowers I've received. Lucky girl X**

Truly, I could have opened a florist with the number of blooms sent my way, as news spread that I was undergoing treatment.

I borrowed vases from neighbours to save buying, as I knew that never again would I receive quite so many bouquets. Even a particularly good Valentine's Day would fail to colour the house in quite such a fashion.

I cherished every card and gift received, and wept many tears over messages sent by friends – some of whom I hadn't seen for years. Experiences like this one build bridges, and over the next few months I would re ignite the flames of friendship with some very special people I should never have let go from my life in the first place ...

**Feel okay but tired at times. Just need to lie down**
**and sleep which is most unlike me! Sonja X**

I am a person who exudes energy from every pore. In my pre-cancer life, I was teaching drama three days a week, writing theatre reviews, directing 80 children at a time in Aberdeen's Scout Gang Show, as well as running my own little darlings between their hobbies as is the wont of every mum.

Chemotherapy would have had a challenge flooring me – but it did succeed where many others have failed. It managed to slow me down a little …

For a while, I stopped everything, deciding that the best action was to keep any energy I had for my own children. I had also been advised to stay away from crowds of strangers, as my immunity had been blitzed by the chemotherapy drugs, so theatre trips and teaching became highly dangerous pastimes to be avoided at all costs.

I am indebted, however, to my friends at the Gang Show, who, realising how important it was for me to have a creative outlet, kept me involved from afar, and left the door open so that I could rejoin rehearsals for the show once I got used to the chemo routine. Gang Show gave me the chance to be 'just Sonja' for a few hours every week – and some much needed down time from the medical world in which I was by now firmly embedded.

**Hi Heidi, Feeling okay, but sore mouth. Just resistance getting low I suppose. Not pleasant but not unexpected either. Lots of love Sonja X**

After five days, the side effects of chemotherapy began. I'd had a strange metallic taste ever since the drugs were administered, and spent the week eating as though trying to combat morning sickness...

Ginger beer, fruit, ice lollies, herbal tea – anything strong tasting and savoury went down a treat. Other than strange dietary habits, however, nothing much changed.

Until the weekend…. The children had gone to Lesley's while the dads played golf and I lay in bed feeling decidedly sorry for myself.

I had the start of a cold sore, and inside my mouth looked like it had been pebble dashed by a cowboy builder and then white washed to cover the cracks. It was sore too – ulcers on my tongue which burned when I ate, and blistering round my lips. The whole look was decidedly unattractive, I felt.

Thankfully I had to go and collect the children – I say thankfully, because if I hadn't, I may well have spent the next four months lying in bed, waiting for the fog to pass. Instead, I got up, gargled with the paint-stripper style mouth wash donated to my cause by the hospital, dabbed on some old cold sore cream which I found languishing in the back of the medicine cabinet, and got dressed.

My short walk round to Lesley's in the late Autumn sunshine made the world a far brighter place. Sipping tea with her while the children played happily in the garden renewed my resolve...

I could lie down and let this beat me, or I could run towards the finishing line, face up to the sun, laughing all the way... Of course, I chose the latter ...

**Keep smiling. You're doing fabulously.
We're so proud of you ... Caroline X**

# Gavin's Story

## Direction by Proxy

When I heard about Sonj's illness I think I reacted by trying to ignore it - ie look for the nearest sandpit and bury my head in it. A reaction I must admit I was not very proud of. I suppose I thought 'yeah she has cancer but she'll be fine', almost treating it like she had a bad cold or the flu!!

It was others around me that gave me the reality check I needed. In the early days people were asking me how she was, how she was coping, how she was feeling and I honestly couldn't tell them because I had been avoiding her and the truth. I soon realised the enormity of what she was going through and knew I should be providing support for her. So what could I do to help?

As you will gather from reading this book, Sonj is not short of a friend!! But my friendship with her was through am-dram and more recently working together to direct Aberdeen Gang Show. I thought this coming year's show 2009 would see Sonj taking a back seat as she would be going through chemo at the time of the bulk of rehearsals, but no, it seemed she had another trick up her sleeve.

What is the saying? "The show must go on". How true that was in Sonj's case. With rehearsals in full swing it was decided that she would work out movement for some of the big company dance numbers, meet me to explain her thoughts and I would go to rehearsals to teach it.

We decided to meet somewhere there wouldn't be lots of people to reduce the risk of her contracting any infection......so Starbucks it was (chuckle).

It was a hoot, imagine the scene. Both of us with our scripts out, me franticly taking notes. Sonj giving little demo's (I hasten to add I didn't copy. After all, we didn't want to get chucked out) and also talking like there was no tomorrow because we needed to catch up on all the gossip!

Even during our meets it was hard to believe Sonj was ill. I suppose the only real sign was the loss of her natural 'blonde' hair.

As she grew stronger our Starbucks meets stopped as she returned to rehearsals and brought the show to the stage. They were a laugh at the time.

Sonj you are truly an inspiration to all. Thanks chum.

# Chapter 12

**Hope you have a great time at Fiona's. Millie and Ed X**

Fiona has always prided herself in being younger than me – not noticeably but enough to have been a constant source of fun between us. Each time I've introduced her as my oldest friend – we've known each other since we were first introduced at dance class when we were four years old – she's jumped in quickly with – "Yes, I am Sonja's oldest friend – but I'm still younger than her!"

The weekend before my second chemo, and six months after my big 4-0 celebration, she was having a party in London to which I had been invited.

When my cancer was diagnosed, I resigned myself to miss it – my oldest and closest friend's birthday and I wouldn't be there.

It did prey on my mind though – I felt pretty good, normal even. Was there really a reason I couldn't travel?

I asked Val – and she fed me the words which I clung onto and made my personal motto - 'If you feel you can Sonja, just do it.'

**Have a ball in London. Enjoy every minute.
Rachel, my sister-in-law X**

We did have a ball that weekend in London. Graham and I jetted off to the capital, booked to see the musical Wicked in the West End – a show I'd been desperate to see for years, and I'm embarrassed to say blubbed all the way through with the sheer emotional impact of the life-changing last few weeks – and then joined Fiona as her 'much-loved oldest friend' – in length of friendship only – at her fabulous 40th birthday party.

> **Thank you so much for coming. It was very special and lovely having you there. Take care. Lots and lots of love Fiona X**

That weekend stands out in my memory partly because it was so much fun, but also because it was a turning point - during those days in the capital, I transformed myself into Red Sonja.

My hair had been coming out in handfuls for the week running up to my London trip... even having a shower was a distressing prospect, knowing I would have to clear the plughole afterwards of my cherished locks.

I stood chatting to friends in the street, while handfuls of hair fell onto my coat. I went to book group and had to clear the chair of swathes of blonde locks as I got up to leave at the end of the evening.

When my ante natal class friend Karen said 'It's not looking too bad – maybe you won't lose all your hair', I chose to demonstrate how it was coming out by running my hands through it. I don't know which of us was more shocked when I was left holding two handfuls of the blonde stuff and wiping away the tears...

So I took the bull by the horns, called Erica for moral support and booked myself in for a haircut.

The plan was to get it shaved and put my wig straight on, no messing - but Kirsteen, who has been cutting mine and the childrens' hair for years, said she couldn't do it. It was too big an ask ...

And so she turned me away from the mirror and gave me a short, elfin look, just like Matthew's and easy to keep – which it was, for all of two days.

Kirsteen confessed to Erica recently that after she cut my hair that day, she went into the back office and cried. I'm afraid to say I went home and did the same ...

> **How's the new hairstyle? Karen X**

> **Get your wig on asap – it's fab! Julie XX**

The underground stations in London are very windy places. I had forgotten that … until I went with my hair in a precarious state. By the time I got to Fiona's it was, as the old Gang Show joke goes, 'Red Indian Style' – Apache…

I chose to wear my wig for the first time in public, as it were, at Fiona's big night out. I knew just a handful of people there, so I figured it gave me the chance to get comfortable with it before facing those who knew me well back home.

At that point, I felt everybody would know I was wearing a wig … because I could feel it, knew it was there, saw myself without it, I couldn't believe that others wouldn't see through the manmade hair to my quickly depleting locks below.

But you know what? They didn't… I had conversations with people and they never once took their eyes off my face to take in my new look. They weren't trying to work out what looked wrong about me, they didn't even know that I looked different – no one but Graham and the children ever saw me with a bald head, and so the illusion worked.

Every time I went out, I looked as though I had just left the hairdresser. I was stylish, beautiful, with catwalk-ready hair shining through the greyest and rainiest of days. I looked and felt fabulous, and with fabulous comes strength and confidence.

From that night on, I wore my wig constantly for six months, only taking it off at bedtime to put on a woolly hat – well, it was cold on those Aberdeen winter nights.

At night, Graham and I lay side by side – his follicly challenged head next to mine, and we laughed … well what else can you do when you are suddenly as bald as the husband you have spent 12 years teasing about his gradually depleting thatch?

When Graham promised to love me 'in sickness and in health' more than a decade before, he had no idea he would be tested so soon …

Three weeks after my first chemo, and the day before my second, Graham shaved my head using his clippers. My heart – and his too, broke over those few bits of fluff left in the shower…

**Wear your wig with pride as you look totally amazing. I am still so inspired by your positivity. You're a star! Love Rachel X**

# Chapter 13

Before every chemotherapy session, I had a date with my oncologist. At first, I thought I was checking in for a run-of-the-mill blood test – and imagined I'd squeeze in a coffee date alongside, just to make the afternoon a little more pleasurable.

Knowing it could work out quite nicely as a social occasion, I asked Sandy (who has always claimed to work in the hospital art gallery) to join me – see how seriously I took these hospital appointments?

Anyway, as is usual in the medical world, things didn't turn out quite as planned, as Sandy chose to outline in great detail on Facebook afterwards to the amusement of our friends…

I'll leave it to her to describe that hospital visit in her own inimitable way:

## Mrs Bling and the Hospital Visit

*"Obviously I spend a lot of time at the hospital installing art, so maybe that is why Mrs Bling thought I might be a suitable companion for her visit to have a blood test. Talk about us both being lulled into a false sense of security.*

*I had just settled down happily with a back copy of Heat magazine, when I am summoned to 'Come on through'. Mmmm, methinks. I didn't know Mrs Bling was squeamish with needles. But hey ho, I don't mind if she wants to wring my hand.*

*Instead, my hand is clapped and wrung by a youngish male doctor, who is giving ME the once over. WELL! But this was mild compared to the twice over he gave Mrs Bling!*

*We were ushered into his domain and with no forewarning, he says to Sonja 'Take your clobber off'." (I don't remember him phrasing it quite like that, but Sandy often knows better ...)*

"Mrs Bling, with her usual style and aplomb immediately starts to de-robe – sans screen. And I mean de-robe. I know layering is in fashion, but you would think Sonja had been having a spell in the North Pole, without central heating, rather than a mild Aberdeen Autumn, by the amount of clothes she had on... While undertaking this mini strip, she clocks her black bra, and with a girlie laugh, says 'Oooh, a black bra under a white shirt'.

By this stage, the doctor (who is obviously used to dealing with over 60-year-olds) looks slightly flustered and then he, with a swirl, flings black bra onto nearby chair, exclaiming 'get rid of that'. WELL, I am nearly falling off my chair and am about to suggest that some sort of decorum must be maintained, but instead manage to just stick to my raised eyebrow expression when he lunges in to start his fiddling!

You would think Mrs Bling was on a sunny nudist beach the way her arms were casually flung back, and all the while Doctor is tittering (excuse the bad pun), measuring and probing and saying things like 'How many centimetres?' ('And what business is that of yours?' I nearly interjected) but then fortunately the re-layering began. Whew.

Dragged myself mentally back onto the chair and gathered my wits about me as Sonja was completely flummoxing the doctor with conversation about the merits of a different hair colour. She then began using that tone (you know the one she uses when she wants you to have the kids and she knows you are resisting just that a little bit) in answer to his perfectly reasonable questions; "Well no, I really can't come in on Friday, I am having my hair done"... pause... doctor (in a bewildered tone) "Can you come in Monday?"... "Well no, I can't, I am off to London for a three-day party"... Doctor, in a slightly apprehensive tone: "Three days of partying in London?" Sonja – "Yes, you see my friend is turning 40 etc etc." Doctor ( looking mildly panicked and in a small voice) "Tomorrow any good for you?"... pause.... "Well yes, I could fit you in tomorrow between my pre-booked shopping trip and my coffee in the afternoon at 2pm..." pause....

Needless to say doctor meekly filled in the required forms and off we trotted with peals of laughter down the corridor and obviously with all NHS protocol gone to pot... this really will not do... I am trying to portray myself as a serious player within the hospital environment ... might just have to nick Mrs Bling's wig for next visit..."

**I'm wearing my wig – and through another chemo! Still looking glamorous! Sonja X**

**You do look glamorous in your wig! Glad to hear you've got through another one. Tick them off! Hope you're not too tired after the hectic weekend. Take care, Fiona X**

And so the cycle begins again ... Erica came with me to my second chemo, and by this time, I'd read and heard all the tips and was more prepared...

To combat nausea, take ginger. Tick, note to self, pack ginger beer.

To help with mouth ulcers, drink pineapple juice. Tick, done.

To make session bearable, bring celebrity mags and a friend, demanding they bring you a nice present to thank you for the privilege of spending an afternoon at the ward with you.

Erica came up trumps on all counts – she even brought a card which made me cry ... "To my wonderfully brave big sister. Step two ... we're nearly halfway there. Keep sparkling!"

I was practically back to normal when I went to the ward that day, armed with all the goodies deemed necessary to come through chemo still smiling.

The instant the drugs were administered, however, the metallic taste returned, driving me to another fortnight of ginger tea and salty pretzels.

It's strange how your body knows exactly what to do ... you just have to learn to listen.

**Nasty taste? Have some pineapple – failing that – gin! Gav**

Losing my hair was a massive ordeal, and to this day stands out as being one of the lowest points of the whole cancer treatment process.

It's not that I'm vain, it's just that I care how I look – let's face it, doesn't every woman get a certain amount of confidence from knowing they've made an effort?

As if sent by my fairy godmother, therefore, a treat arose that put the sparkle back in my step – The Look Good Feel Better workshop ...

Organised by the hospital, and supported by the world's leading cosmetic houses, these workshops are open to all going through Breast Cancer treatment.

And so it came to pass that I joined 15 women in a small room at the hospital, sharing mirrors and cancer stories, all the while learning how to disguise the ravages of chemo and pursue life without the telltale signs of treatment.

While we rubbed, brushed and moisturised, we chatted and laughed, women of many ages and backgrounds bonding over the shared experience of battling cancer. Each coping in our own way, strong and focussed - the past already behind us and reinventing ourselves for the present.

The future ... well, that was too far away to think about. At this stage, I wasn't sure if I'd ever think about the future again ...

**Radiotherapist Martin Rudge, who I interviewed later in this book, was around for the launch of the Look Good Feel Better Project.**

**He says of it:**

"The Look Good Feel Better project is brilliant, the number of women who get such a buzz out of it. I was asked to go along and help launch it, and as a bloke in a room full of beauticians – I could see why it was important to women. It's all about projecting an image. For women, image is so important, and if they lose that, they lose part of themselves.

"By letting women get together and chat, and learn about keeping themselves looking great and healthy throughout their breast cancer treatment, you're giving them the tools to remain happy too."

# Chapter 14

**I always believed that Gang Show needed to be constant for you, to dip in and out as you could. However, your positive reaction to situations meant that everything moved on in time and we reached the end of the journey with an excellent show ...**
**Ian Dow, Gang Show Convener and Friend**

It's not as if Gang Show has been just a passing phase in my life. I joined the Gang when I became a Venture Scout at the age of 15, and took on the choreographer's mantle when I was 21.

By 23, I was directing and choreographing the entire show, and apart from a couple of years when I had the children, I have been involved in the production team for over 15 years. Last year I was rewarded for my efforts with a Medal of Merit for my services to Scouting ... Pretty special by all accounts...

Throughout those 25 years, Ian Dow has been a friend and ally, picking me up when I was struggling and clipping my wings when I took on too much – as is often my way.

Many other hobbies fell by the wayside when undergoing chemotherapy, but Gang Show ... well, my life felt empty without it.

And so I returned. Just before going back for my third chemotherapy session, I made Gang Show my special treat for the weekend, and arrived, new look at the ready, to see if I still 'had it' as far as the Gang were concerned.

I walked in, almost shyly, sure 'the Gang' wouldn't recognise or remember me – they are kids after all, and one adult is very much like another for most teenagers.

As I took in their surprised, happy faces, I realised that they were rising to their feet, clapping, cheering, relieved that I looked normal, I was still there – under the red wig – I was still the Sonja who would rally the troops and pull the show together.

Over the next few months, I did what I could, turned up when I was able, and somehow, as a team, we produced the best Gang Show ever seen on Aberdeen's stage … and the happiest, most fulfilled woman ever to fight breast cancer.

I had found my secret weapon – and once again, I used it in style…

**My son took part in his first Gang Show this year and had so much fun. I was impressed with the cast, the show in general and in particular Sonja for pulling this together while going through her treatment. I know well how much chemotherapy takes out of you, but any time I picked up from rehearsals or helped at the show, Sonja was smiling… a real inspiration.**
**Gang Show Mum**

Skerry became my third chemo buddy. Reaching the halfway point was definitely a landmark. I knew what I was doing, how I would feel, and I started giving advice to newcomers to the ward, just as others had to me a couple of months before.

It was during this third visit that I started to notice the chemotherapy ward. Paint peeling off the walls, functional wipe-clean chairs and no privacy, even if you needed it. In fact, it was Skerry who pointed out that the chemotherapy ward had all the charm and homeliness of an Old Folk's Home – only most of us were there 40 years' too soon… At that point a spark was ignited, which burned slowly through to January, when I decided to do something about it…

**Halfway? Good going girl! Hope you're feeling more like yourself soon… Sarah, neighbour and friend X**

The aftermath of the third chemotherapy session wasn't quite the textbook case to which I had become accustomed. In the middle of the night afterwards, I was sick for the first time.

Didn't take the anti sickness drugs soon enough, I imagine – tried to be a superhero and fell flat on my face most definitely, but it wasn't pleasant. Thankfully however, it's the one and only time it happened – and I know I had been getting complacent with the ease I was sailing through the whole experience. I mean, some people have this (and far worse) every time ...

And 10 years ago, well let's face it, the third session of chemotherapy would have been a far harder place to be. ...

**Oh love! You are being so brilliant about all this. I hope you feel better soon. Keep fighting XX Fiona**

**Hi Soggs, Hope you're feeling a bit better today. That must be you halfway there. Keep well, Keith X**

# Message from fellow Pink Lady Nikki

Nikki, who was diagnosed with breast cancer in 2006, has been a constant source of support to me over the last year. Her many tips got me through chemotherapy and radiotherapy and I've included many of them in the Doing It With Bling On Tips at the end of this book. Nikki wrote to me before the Bling Fling, explaining a little about her own breast cancer journey:

"I'm so looking forward to taking part in the Bling Fling, along with my team 'Buddies Out On Bling Sunday (BOOBS)!...

I was diagnosed with breast cancer in November 2006. Of course I was gutted but decided I would get through the journey that lay ahead. I always remained very positive and tried to remain cheery and keep busy.

After my mastectomy, six months of chemotherapy and six weeks of radiotherapy, I realised just how amazing my family and friends and work mates had been. I'd say to anyone who has to deal with such news, always to remain positive – it really helps.

My 'chemo bud', my friend Lainey, was my rock. She arranged all her days off so she could attend my chemo visits. We laughed, chatted, ate and just chilled. I'd say 'Always have a chemo bud!'

The hospital staff are amazing and soon became very important people in my life. I also wore a cold cap, which amazingly let me keep my hair throughout my treatment. It's pretty amazing, although at -25 it is very cold, but very worthwhile nonetheless.

When I heard about Sonja I was very upset and we got in touch – I sent her positive vibes and a few tips via Facebook.

We have kept in touch and when she told me about the Bling Fling, I was delighted as it's on my 44th birthday.

I think it's amazing that she's organised such a wonderful event. I'm delighted to help raise funds for the ward where I received so much care and visited so often.

Sonja – a total inspiration to us all, Let's have a ball at the Bling Fling!

## Chapter 15

**Hope you get good news this am. Thinking about you. Sorry I can't be there. Erica X**

Celebration at the halfway point wasn't just confined to ticking another box on the calendar.

Yes, I had three sessions under my belt and I knew I was coping with the whole routine... but there was another big question to be answered... was it working?

The oncologist wasn't sure ... he did his usual measuring trick, humming and hawing over my breast all the while using a ruler type gadget to measure 'the lump', which by now I couldn't feel...

To my shock, however, he declared that it was still there, it was measuring the same as it had been at the beginning, and he broke it to me none too gently that the chemotherapy may not be working. Worse, he might have to change the drugs concoction for the next part of treatment, and worse still, I would need another four doses to shrink it properly ... oh no, no, no, no, no ... my fighting spirit took a pounding with this news...

But as always, and with Val's amazing commitment to my case, I got back into the ring, and waited for the next mammogram and ultrasound appointment – booked just before my fourth chemotherapy dose to give the drugs maximum chance to do their stuff...

More photographs of my relatively unglamorous breasts? I was starting to feel that my birthday suit had been photographed more often than a Page 3 girl's.

For this modelling assignment, I enlisted the support of Lesley and her lovely laugh once more and headed for the out-patients X-ray department of Aberdeen Royal Infirmary. By this time, I knew the best parking spaces, staff canteen and was fully versed with the short cut through the laundry (shown to me by Sandy, and followed that day by Lesley and I, giggling like school girls who suspected they were about to be caught out and dragged screaming in front of the headmaster.)

When asked to prepare myself for the tests, you'll be glad to know that by this time I had learned from the time-consuming strip tease experience of Sandy's observation, and dressed in clothes I knew could easily be removed, leaving my wig intact.

**Keeping fingers and toes crossed for you! Sarah X**

As Lesley caught up on one of the magazines she hadn't yet got round to reading – in those days, she had read every bit of print lying around every ward and clinic in the hospital, and was quoting celebrity gossip at me ad nauseum – I bared my all for another barrage of tests...

Those of you who have yet to know the charm of the mammogram machine, count yourself lucky. This is how it is...

You stand, naked from the waist up, while some nurse with freezing hands manhandles your boob into position onto an even colder plate.

"Stand back ... towards me ... left a bit ... right a bit.... There.... Now lean forward ... no don't take your heels off the floor ... oh ... no ... that's a bit off ... okay ... don't worry ... stand back ... right ... let's try again."

When finally your breast is in position, pop stud sticker in place to mark your nipple (very Heath Robinson), a top plate comes down to clamp you in place. Think George Formby grill on steroids and you get the general idea.

Now imagine this ... the plate squeezes down ... and down ... and down... until you can't take it any longer ... your boobs are going to burst.... they'll explode all over the room ... aaaaaaaaaahhhhhh...

the pain ..... a sudden click ... it releases.... And you feel the relief flooding through ...

It's over ... until the next time. Because when you have cancer, you know there is always a mammogram waiting for you before the next hurdle...

Ultrasound, on the other hand, is a breeze – especially this one, when the news was so good.

The last time I'd had good news at an ultra sound scan was when I was pregnant. Two tiny arms.... Two tiny legs... a heart beating bravely in the blob of life growing with me ... all present and correct, sir!

With this scan, it was what they didn't find that brought such good news... Because the radiographer looked, and she struggled, and she looked, and she went back to the original x-rays, and she looked ... and finally, she found it, a tiny trace of what had been there before.

The tumour ... barely there... a shadow of its former self ... the chemotherapy was working...

> **I got the best news today ... the tumour has shrunk so much they had to put a marker in!! Sonja**

> **Am so delighted for you and feel positive some of that must be down to your amazing attitude. You have been absolutely inspiring. Kay, book group friend X**

> **Wow, that is amazing. It is fantastic to hear the good news. Prayers have definitely been answered. Tracey, friend X**

> **That's brilliant news. Chemo must be working wonders! Callum, Gang Show Musical Director X**

# Chapter 16

**You may be there already, but hope this afternoon's session goes ok X Skerry**

By the time I got to the third week after chemotherapy, each time I was feeling well again ... no sore mouth, no strange metallic taste. Even my energy levels were returning to normal. It's amazing how much of this stuff your body can take and still comes back smiling...

Knowing you will recover doesn't make it any easier to go through the endurance test each time, however, and this is where the chemo buddy scheme really kicked in. A new friend with me every three weeks kept the chore from becoming monotonous or traumatic – it distracted me from the awfulness of what was to come. I heard a whole new set of problems, stories and gossip – with each friend putting the world to rights while the nurses injected the poison through my poor unsuspecting veins. (Actually, I think they were starting to suspect something was going on, as they shrunk out of reach every time the nurse went near them to administer the final doses)

My taste buds were also beginning to get wise to the fresh pineapple and ginger, making me gag as I tried to pack them away in a futile attempt to curb the strange sensations in my mouth and stomach.

The laughs, however, which made it all the more bearable, were still very much in evidence – for the fourth session, supplied by the Queen of Laughter herself, Lesley, whose peals of joy made the whole ward seem an altogether more sparkling place.

**Another one down! Soon be finished ... Sonja**

**Roll on that day! Jillian, college friend**

**Good for you! It's done and it's doing the trick. Just keep gritting the teeth. Ailsa, neighbour X**

**You are supersonic – well done! Jill, Book group friend**

The best thing about my final three chemotherapy sessions was the time of year in which they took place. Like all families, our calendar is filled to bursting in November, December and January, and my body processing heavy doses of poisonous drugs made no difference to ours.

Although I have to confess that Bonfire night at my brother Keith's after my fourth session brought its own hazards...

Like the London underground presents a nightmare for precarious hair, Keith's magnificent bonfire, which gets bigger each year (I'm sure this one could be seen from outer space) was particularly scary for little ol' wig-wearer me.

As the fire shot sparks high into the sky above his family home, and my nieces and nephews closed in around me with out-of-control sparklers, which they threw in my direction as the sparks got dangerously close to their tiny hands, I felt ... um, how shall I say this? .... Vulnerable seems like an understatement... Shit scared is probably more accurate.

One spark on my beautiful red (but totally man-made) locks would cause chaos – the nylon hair melting and sticking to my by now smooth-as-a-baby's-bottom scalp.

So I sat, as far from the fire as possible, hat pulled down over my beautiful coiffure, and watched ... and waited ... willing the day that I could enjoy the sensation of the wind in my hair, and the heat of the fire in my face, once more.

> **You continue to inspire me with how you deal with all of this. You are two thirds of the way through. Well done you! Such great news that it is working so well and shrinking the tumour so dramatically. Rachel**

> **Let's take some bubbly to the last one! Only two more… Well done you! Janine**

No sooner was Guy Fawkes done and dusted, than my favourite time of year came a-knocking.

All right, I confess, I love Christmas. Even before I had kids I loved it … and now, the children give me an excuse to love it more.

I can't get enough of the decorations, coal fires, candles, shopping, Christmas food … you name it. Except this year was different…

I did decorate the house, early in December, during my feelgood third week. Presents were bought online or early in the morning to avoid crowds – I stayed away from bugs at all costs during this particularly bug-ridden time of year, knowing that my body was no longer able to fight them off.

Christmas food lost its sparkle for me. The sweet things I usually enjoy as a guilt-free indulgence during the festive season, played havoc with my mouth, bringing it out in ulcers, and my tongue rubbed itself raw at times with sugar overload.

I did, however, develop a taste for mulled wine and savoury snacks – and it being Christmas, as well as everyone feeling sorry for me, cut me the slack to have plenty of both…

> **How are you doing? Hope you are resting enough at this mad time of year. Thinking of you, Julie X**

I also found time to rest (not usual for me amidst the enjoyable chaos that Christmas usually involves) … but rest I did, lulled into relaxation while sitting in a darkened room eating popcorn. This lovely girly treat took place mid-December, when Lesley and I booked tickets alongside all the OAPs and Nursing Home Bus Tours to see Bing Crosby's White Christmas, digitally remastered and showing at one of Aberdeen's biggest cinema houses.

What an experience ... a daytime jaunt to the cinema, sitting with groups of nostalgic old ladies sharing sandwiches and yearning for the good old days. Daytime cinema visits are surely one of life's ultimate indulgences – an indulgence we never would have discovered without breast cancer treatment.

**Merry Christmas to all my wonderful friends ... Sonja X**

## Lesley's Story

Let me just start by saying Sonja has been remarkable in how she has coped with this terrible time in her life. Would we all cope so well? I hope I never have to find out.

What I do know is that I watched her, and tried to help her along the way of this long and terrible journey that is called cancer. She is a great friend, she is such fun to be with and we have shared many happy times despite the sometimes dark days of her battle. What I tried to do for her, and this is a reflection of my own personality, was just to be there for her and her family.

I am a practical beast and am wary of over-emotionality and sentimentality……in this way, Sonja and I are a little different. She is exuberance itself and embraces life to the full. This is her way of living and she does it so well. I have to say I didn't think of bringing a present to the chemo session I attended with her, I haven't lavished flowers on her, but I would like to think that it is what I have done is what she will remember….the several visits to the hospital, helping to organise the Bling Fling, having the kids for tea or a sleepover…. all of which have been a pleasure and have brought me on my own journey of sorts.

And, of all the hard things I have had to do for Sonja, is accompany her on trips to the cinema…and in the middle of the day…what a drag! No, what a joy it was! What of these midday cinema trips do I remember most?

I will, of course, always remember seeing Star Trek. There I was lusting over Captain Kirk when Sonja said he looked very much like the husband of a friend of ours. That definitely killed the mood!

Or Bride Wars where we laughed our socks off? Last Chance Harvey, starring Dustin Hoffman and Emma Thompson, was delicious and we were left speechless at how this couple communicated and shared so well and led to a great discussion about relationships.

But overall, the best, indulgent trip to the cinema was to see White Christmas. There we were, two lovely ladies in our early forties, surrounded by a whole cinema full of awe-struck pensioners as we watched the digitally-enhanced version of the film. It was glorious, magnificent and bolstered us up, letting us capture the wonderful essence of Christmas despite the huge challenges Sonja was facing.

We all have to face our own mortality. Sonja has had to do it head-on. By helping her through this amazingly difficult time, I feel I've had to face this issue myself, albeit in a far less significant way. What would I do, how would I react? Those questions went through my head so many times.

Sadly, my father-in-law died of prostate cancer whilst Sonja was in the midst of her struggle and seeing him in the last throes of life was heartbreaking.

What a year it has been. But I have learnt a lot and I thank Sonja for allowing me to help her fight, and beat, the biggest challenge of her life!

# Chapter 17

**Hope today goes fine doll. Skerry X**

My fifth blast started with a laugh – at the expense of the hospital car parking system...

Julie, who had the special privilege of being my festive chemo buddy, collected me from town where I had spent the morning shopping and 'doing lunch' with mum and Erica. This is distraction policy at its best – keeping myself busy so that there is no time to think about the monster looming in my path has been the saving grace throughout my cancer journey.

That mid-December day, Julie arrived, dressed up to the nines as instructed, and brandishing mince pies and a fully wrapped Christmas present which she threw into my lap with an explanatory 'It's just something small – should make you laugh! You could always use it to take your mind off things this afternoon.'

Laugh was exactly what I did – peals of it as I opened the beautifully wrapped gift to reveal a Design Your Own Beaver kit.

Iron filings and a magnet squeezed into a plastic frame, just like in Christmases of old, kept me going as I came up with intricate designs to try out when mine grew back... yes, the fact that I was somewhat follicly challenged in that department seemed like the funniest thing in the world just at that moment.

Julie didn't know, hadn't twigged somehow, that the drugs aren't selective in any way – arms, nasal hairs, legs, eyebrows, lashes, other bits, you name it. Where there's hair, they'll do the work of any manic beautician and get the better of it... Well, how would she know? It's not something you would automatically think about is it? If it's any consolation, it took me quite by surprise too... I'm not sure that I ever got over Emma's exclamation as I emerged from the shower; 'Mummy, you look just like me now...' Not really words you want to hear from your gorgeous seven-year-old princess, but cancer does that. Opens conversations you never wanted to have, with people you'd do everything to protect...

Apart from finding my funniest chemo present, Julie also provided me that day with the most fun-packed and memorable journey to the hospital.

Julie drives a very big, very grand jeep complete with private number plates, cruise control and in-built satellite navigation. Not that I'm a gadget lover in any way whatsoever, but this is one cool car, and we felt invincible arriving at the already crowded pre-Christmas car park...

Which is probably why, when we saw the queue – estimated to be at least half an hour to parking time (time we didn't have as we were, as is our prerogative, running late) – we decided to take a risk... live life dangerously as it were. As if at the time I wasn't living dangerously enough...

And so we abandoned our rather grand-looking wheels in the private car park of a nearby office block, and giggled as we crept past the glass doors of the reception area, looking about as guilty as any two women could look in such an everyday situation.

Well, red-handed we certainly were caught when minutes later, we were hauled up by an officious looking receptionist who told us in no uncertain terms that this was a private car park and we would have to move on ... Of course we complied, still snorting with laughter at the fun of it all, only to be caught once again trying to sneak into the main hospital car park from the wrong direction.

Oh it felt good to be rebellious for a while, flouting the rules in our huge bully of a vehicle. When we eventually flashed my appointment card and were shown into the completely legitimate patient parking in the hospital grounds, it seemed somewhat disappointing that our rule-breaking had been unnecessary... but it was fun, and the laughs that ensued kept us going through another onslaught of the hard stuff...

> **Hiya, how did you get on today? Just think, one more to go! Have a good night. See you tomorrow. Lesley**

Christmas, for me, is an excuse to do all the things I'd really want to be doing all year, but can't get away with it without looking a little eccentric.

I remember as a student working as a waitress at a Christmas party in July, and thinking that must be the ultimate in nights out – Christmas at any time of year is my idea of heaven.

And so, chemo or no chemo, I decided to hold a Christmas party for my friends, complete with mulled wine, mince pies and lots of chocolate…. And, in spite of my innate fear of naked flames, I enlisted the help of a candle party hostess to lend some sparkle to the event.

Everyone arrived, blinged up for the festive season and bearing gifts for the raffle table, and we laughed and chatted as the candle wicks depleted and the friendships grew. Old pals caught up, new contacts were made, and the money came rolling in - £100 for Breast Cancer Research from one fun-packed evening of partying.

An idea which had begun in the chemotherapy ward a couple of weeks before started to smoulder that night … by the New Year, it would become a fire, raging within me – a new focus as fundraiser and inspirer was waiting in the wings, ready to envelope me and my group of friends with it.

> **Thanks for a lovely night. Nice to catch up with everyone… You are fab! Jacqui X**

By Christmas week, the metallic taste was starting to wane, the ulcers subsiding and I was re-entering the world once more, able to join the fun of a family Christmas Day.

Our children, the third generation of a performing family – my mum was a dancer and my sisters and I have all been known to tread the boards on occasion in our misspent youth – can't help but seek the limelight every December 25, rehearsing a show for those adults not too full or drunk enough to fall asleep and avoid it.

My battle had become so familiar to the children by December, that my own two starlets and their three cousins took it upon themselves to stage the Breast Cancer Show, fleecing us for cash before every act, holding a raffle for a 'Breast Cancer Bear' and placing every penny into my youngest nephew's piggy bank, to be added to the Candle Party fund once the troops had been entertained.

And so, bloated with Christmas dinner and unable to run, we took our places on the re-arranged sofas to proudly partake in our children's star turns – performed with aplomb by our super-confident brood, and introduced by four-year-old director Lachlan.

Hearing a child of his age speak so candidly and openly about breast cancer is slightly surreal – but in the four months since my cancer was diagnosed, the words and feelings associated with it had become part of the children's language, and were no longer the instigator of tears or sadness. They were matter-of-fact, everyday words that were used without embarrassment or hesitation.

Much as children look to us for reassurance in these matters, so we must look to them for their ease in handling the information. Children absorb news – even of the worst kind. Some worry, some brood, some get angry, some contemplative … but in time, all adjust, regroup and refocus, then carry on with their lives, slightly altered but just as strong as ever they were.

Oh that we could all deal with life with the intuition of our children…

**Happy New Year! May it bring everything you wish for … Sonja X**

These wishes were more for me than for anyone else, if I'm honest. What did I wish for on those 12 strokes of midnight before the world burst into a drunken rendition of Auld Lang Syne? Good health is the easy one … and then there are all the usual things. The things other 40-year-olds wish on themselves and their family. Happiness, success, happiness … and health. Always health … Never before had I been so worried about my health … never before had I had to be.

2009 would be the year I got healthy… the year that I didn't have to worry about my health any more. Well wouldn't it?

# Chapter 18

**See you when I've been zapped! Sonja**
**Just a note to say well done you for getting to the last**
**of the six and handling it all so calmly and fabulously**
**well girl. You are a real inspiration. Skerry X**

We celebrated my last trip to the chemo ward on January 5$^{th}$, 2009, and this time, we did it with bling on. Janine, who was my last ever chemo buddy, offered to bring champagne to begin the celebrations – but I declined. Not like me I know, but knowing from experience that ginger beer would do a better job on the inevitable side effects. The fact that this was my last session would do little to lessen the impact of the drugs on my body – but, it being my last meant that I was in the mood to celebrate – and no amount of the hard stuff would dampen my spirits that I'd reached the first goal on my recovery from breast cancer.

As was often the case, my arrival at the ward – almost on time but not quite – was still too early for the consistently hard worked staff. Janine and I were dispatched to sit in the waiting room and start on the hard work of the next three hours – gleaning gossip from the latest celebrity magazines and eating and drinking our carefully chosen snacks.

Not much reading went on that day, however, as the wheels of my imagination were at work – and fired by Janine's enthusiasm for fundraising, in the next hour we came up with the initial idea that would in time become the biggest, pinkest event Aberdeen had ever seen.

As I looked around at the peeling walls and unadorned windows of the chemotherapy ward, the painters' daughter in me observed that the surroundings were far from the comfortable, calming place it should be. Something in me realised at that point that we could and should do something about it ... bling it up, so to speak.

If we could raise some money, we could leave our mark on the ward, giving it a makeover which would add a little sparkle to all those receiving chemotherapy in our wake.

We may even raise enough to provide magazines and some complementary therapies to make the whole experience a far more bearable prospect.

We spoke at length. To be honest I can't remember who originated what idea. All I can remember is that we came up with the idea for a sponsored walk, a party afterwards, a theme of Tiaras and Trainers – and a possible title.

By the time I was gagging on the last chunk of pineapple I would ever eat, the Bling Fling was born... and my trips to the chemotherapy ward were over.

**All done! Last blast today. Yippee! Have a celebration drink for me tonight. Thanks for helping me get through. Sonja X**

**Well done you. Sometimes we have no choice with the things life throws at us, but you are a star girl – cheers and fantastic. Very happy for you, Jillian X**

The end of chemotherapy marked the finishing line – or at least, the first finishing line of my journey ... The six chemotherapy dates in my diary had been ticked off, the first six blood tests undertaken and passed with flying colours, but what now? Perhaps my hair would instantly grow back? My periods restart – or, god forbid, my menopause?? Maybe I'd have to start shaving my legs? And what's more, I could re emerge into the world in which I used to live – do the things I used to do before I became terrified of flu bugs and strangers sneezing...

Sadly, all the changes chemotherapy renders take far longer to put right than the course of drugs ending... my nose still ran continuously in those winter months, with no hair to catch the drips.

I've never felt more like a nursery child than I did that January while trying to avoid long mummy chats on street corners. Nothing less glamorous than wiping a dripping nose on your coat sleeve I've found, black and fur-trimmed though it most likely is where I'm concerned...

Nothing about my life would return to normal for months, so to celebrate, I did two things – I bought myself a new wig, and planned a girls' weekend away to St Andrews to launch yet another new me. By this time, I was relishing every opportunity to reinvent myself, and charity shops were my little piece of heaven where I could buy other people's forgotten treasures and work them into my already bulging wardrobe...

I decided to treat myself to a new hairstyle – for that, read wig – at the end of January, when I felt I deserved it, having saved enough on hairdresser's bills over the last few follicly challenged months. It was also in my mind that my hair would start growing in eventually, and I should perhaps go for an in-between look. I wouldn't want to wear my wig forever and to go from long and red to short and elfin in one fleeting night might be too much to handle for those around me...

And so, on my own this time, I headed back to Rose at Finishing Touches to seek advice on a new me for the new year - and to see me through to my final reinvention of myself, when I re-emerged in April with the shortest, snappiest (and curliest) haircut I've ever known.

Strangely, I went for the wig that I was drawn to in the first place – and the one which, had the children not accompanied me on that first visit, I would probably have chosen from the outset. A classic bob, in red with blonde highlights, it was the perfect step between wig-wearing and au natural, and filled the intervening months perfectly. It was much admired, gave me the chance to buy some new clothes to complement the chic 1920s look and, I must confess, felt a whole lot more like me.

Long and red was glamorous, different, striking even ... but it was never quite my style, and the new bob which swung when I walked, shone in the sun and never had a hair out of place, was far more akin to the Sonja I used to know... I was back, the chemotherapy was over, and a new target was in my sights...

To celebrate the end of chemotherapy, and to reenergise myself ready for the next step in treatment – the already looming surgeon's knife – I did what the advert says and took a break.

Sandy, Lisa, and Lesley were my travelling partners of choice on this occasion, and together we packed our bags – for most of us, one small suitcase would suffice, for kleptomaniac Sandy (who had recently returned from a trip to India with three large containers full of clothes), no less than three holdalls were necessary to carry her basic essentials for the weekend.

How we laughed as she unpacked blankets, pillows, five outfits (complete with shoes) – yet she still borrowed an outfit of mine as she had 'nothing to wear' at the last minute – and of course, her 1950s swimsuit complete with cone-shaped underwiring which cuts a Madonna-like dash around the swimming pool.

Over that weekend, we hit the charity shops and antique centres, stopping often for girly chats over steaming cups of coffee in the wonderful student haunts around the gorgeous university town of St Andrews, and laughed at the stories and memories of the last few months.

Before bedtime, we gathered on the beds of one of the rooms, drinking wine and chatting and joking as if we were teenage dorm mates telling scary stories after lights out in a girls' school. I felt comfortable and confident with those friends around me to reveal all, and finally stripped myself of my new and already itching wig to sit in my bald loveliness while the girls declared I had 'a nicely shaped head'. Hmmm… good to know on such occasions, I guess.

Lisa was the one friend who couldn't hide her shock when I threw my hair casually to the side and poured myself a glass of wine as a distraction policy. She looked, and I could see her thoughts swimming around behind the mild panic in her eyes.

When I asked her about it, she said: "It's just easy to forget what you've been going through. It's not until now that I realised…" I know exactly what she meant. My whole illusion had worked, and for that I was truly grateful. And now, with chemotherapy behind me, I could let those closest to me into my secret – and as we hugged, and they touched and I laughed at the beauty of my cheek bones (as they described them), I knew that I was among friends…. non judgemental, wonderful friends, who would always be there and see me, only me….always…

## Janine's Story

I still get that sinking feeling every time I think about the day Sonja told me she had found a lump.

The kids had just gone back to school after the summer holidays. I'd missed a couple of calls from Sonja and it was on my mind to phone her when I got THE call.

It just didn't seem possible. For the last few months we had been basking in the glory of memories of a fantastic family holiday together when the only thing we had to worry about was what cocktail we were going to have at noon and what martini we would have before dinner ! Life was good and then suddenly, this. Talk about coming down to earth with a bump.

I immediately jumped in the car and went round to Sonja's. She told me everything that had happened since finding the lump and what was going to happen next.

She was incredibly brave and positive and told me that because I was such a positive person she knew I could help her get through this.

Of course everything was going to be alright I told her. Don't ever think any different. By this time next year this will just be a memory.

I went home feeling a complete fraud. I had lost my beloved mum to breast cancer a few years before and the thought of Sonja going through the same thing was almost too much to bear. I was devastated for her, for how Graham and the kids and her mum and dad must be feeling. I cried all the way home. I was shaking. I tried to phone my husband to tell him but he couldn't understand a word I was saying. And all the time I was so angry because I felt I was being sorry for myself.

I think I was just in shock. After I calmed down I hoped I could be the friend Sonja needed.

Sonja had a plan to fight the disease – to live life to the full - to focus on the positive and never let the cancer control her life. Anyone looking at Sonja would never have known there was anything wrong with her. She had a great range of wigs and hats that made her look great and always did her make up so well that she looked stunning.

Over the next few months we did all the nice things that normal life got in the way of but now we realized the importance of. We had lunch, went for coffee, walks, chatted a lot and had a family weekend away. All through her treatment Sonja stayed well and looked fabulous.

I remember how elated I felt when Sonja said that she felt that the tumour was shrinking.

When a final scan at the end of her chemotherapy confirmed that the tumour had all but disappeared I was just delighted.

I went with Sonja to her last chemotherapy session and despite the depressing surroundings we spent our time laughing and chatting and coming up with the Bling Fling idea that led to us, along with four other friends, raising over £70,000 for breast cancer research at Aberdeen Royal Infirmary and other related services and another local charity supporting children and adults with learning disabilities called Archway.

If there is anything good that can come out of a devastating disease like this it's that it makes you realize who and what is really important in life.

I am so proud of Sonja and glad I can call her my friend. Here's to following dreams and living life to the full - with bling on!

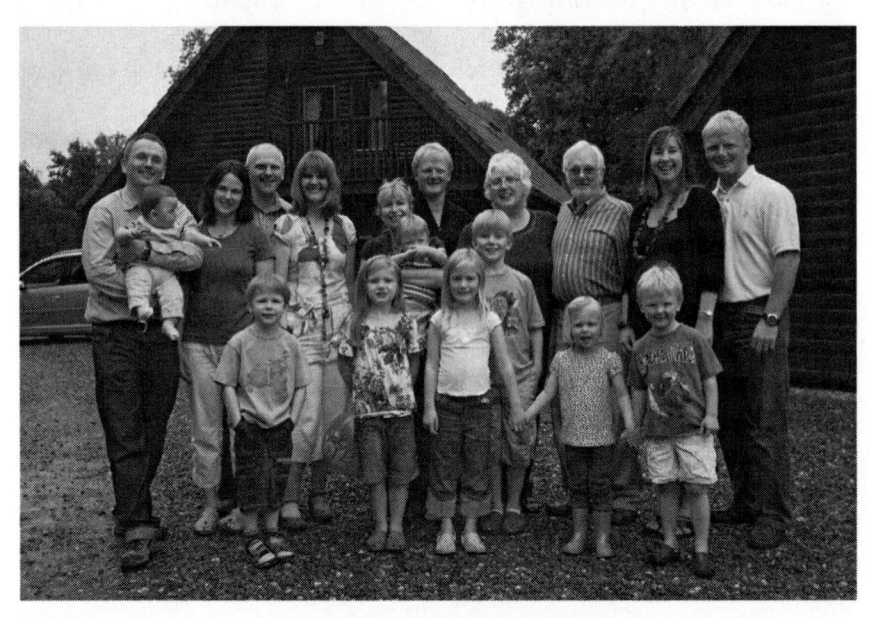

Loch Lomond Read Family Group

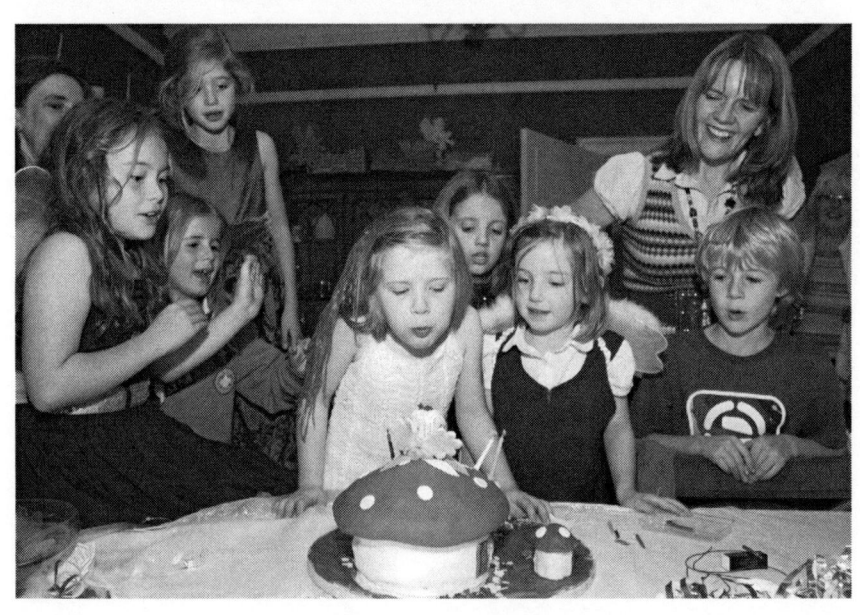

Sonja at Emmas 7th Birthday

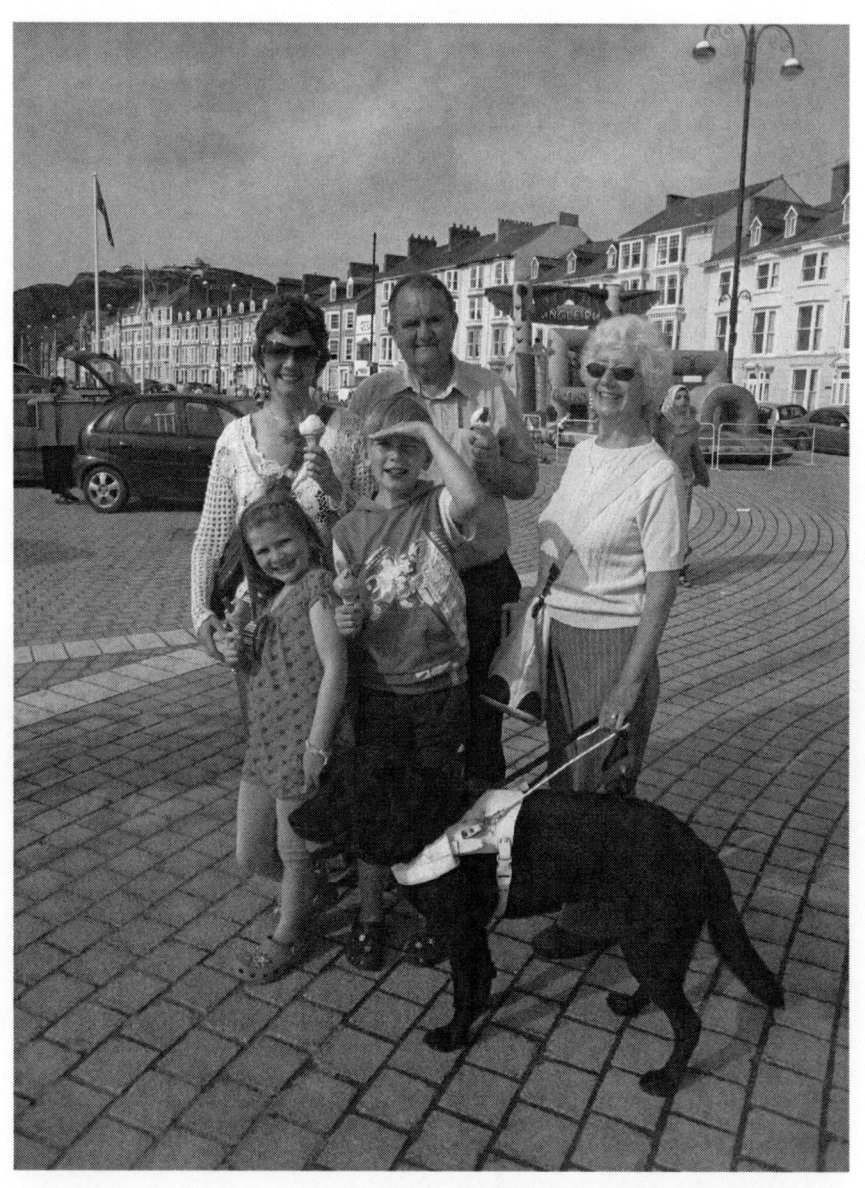

Mum, dad, the kids and guide dog Campbell on holiday in Wales

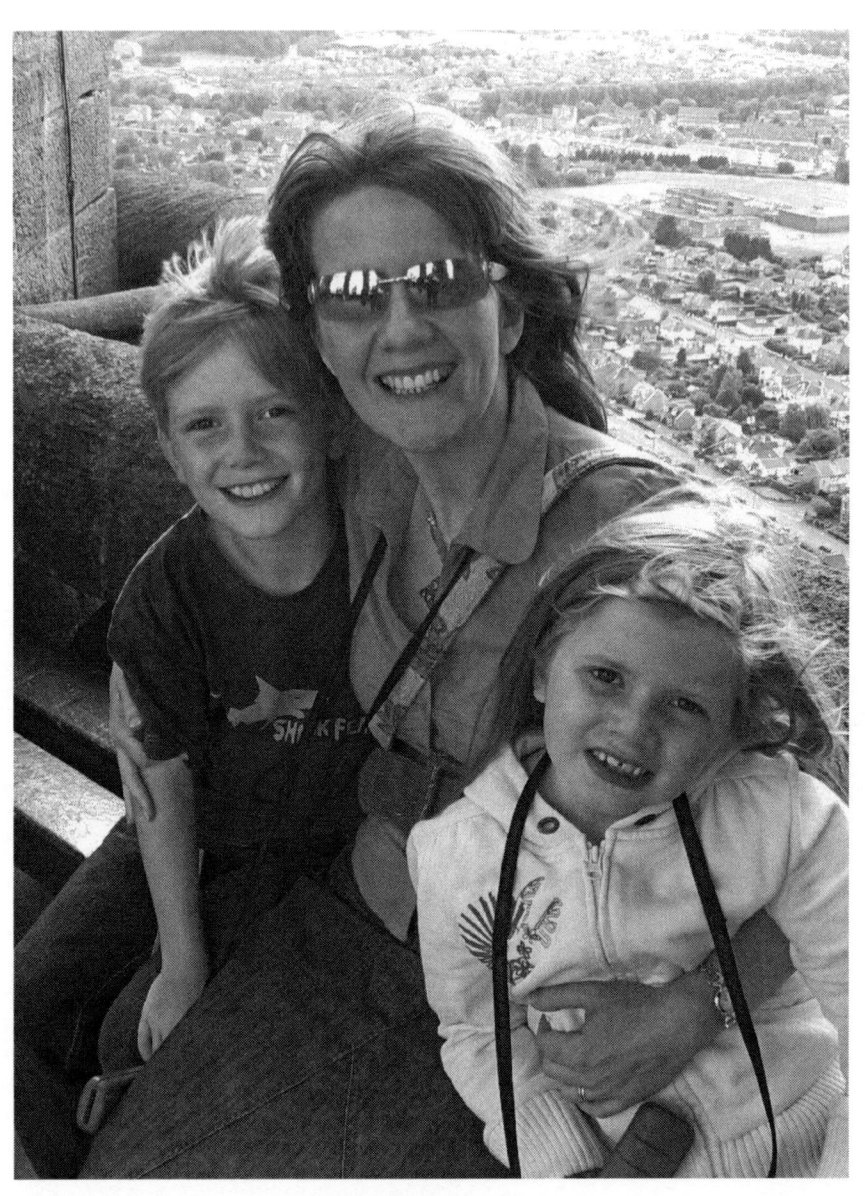

Sonja Kids Wallace Monument

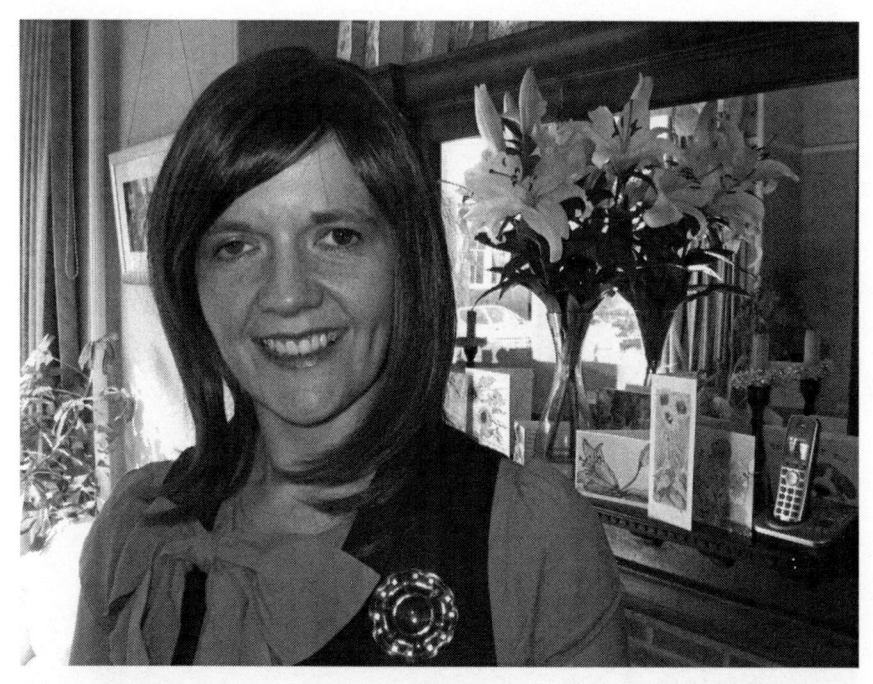

Sonja with wig

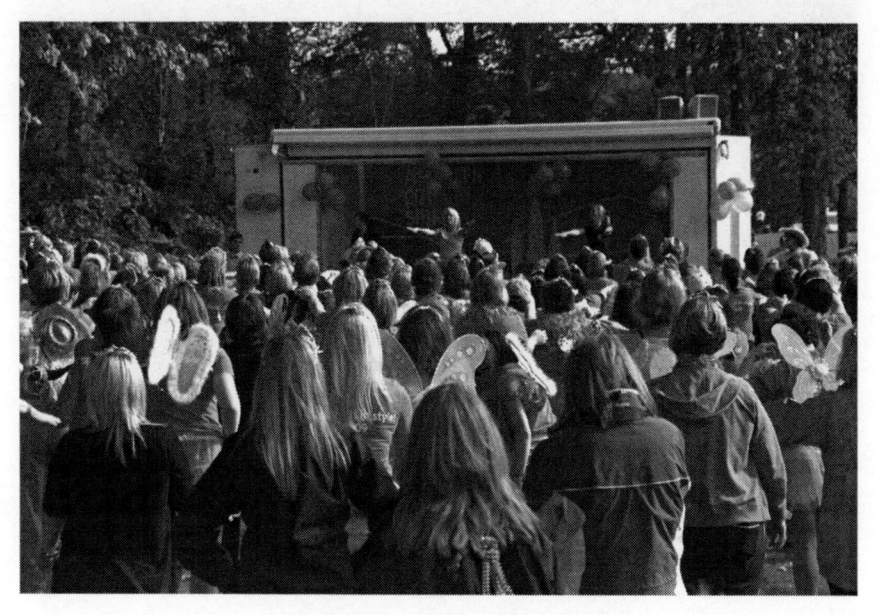

Warming up at the Bling Fling

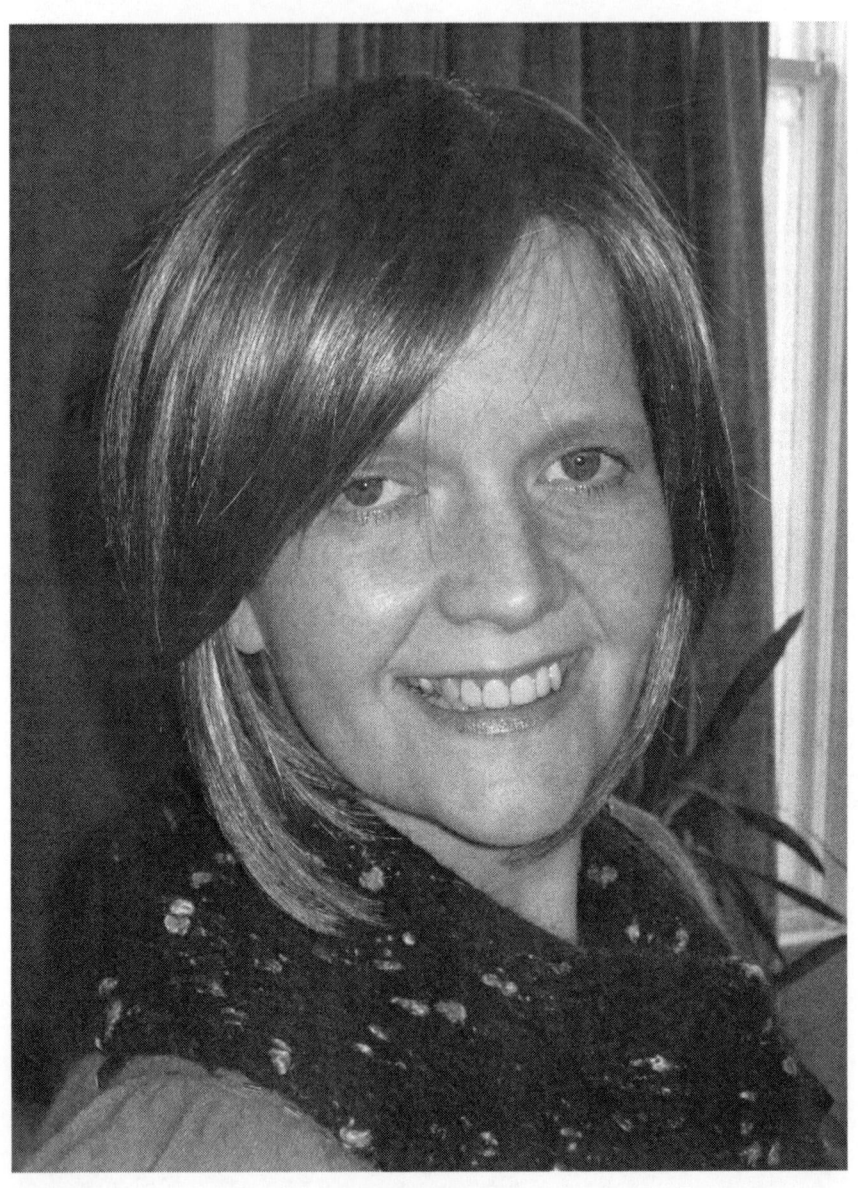

Sonja with wig

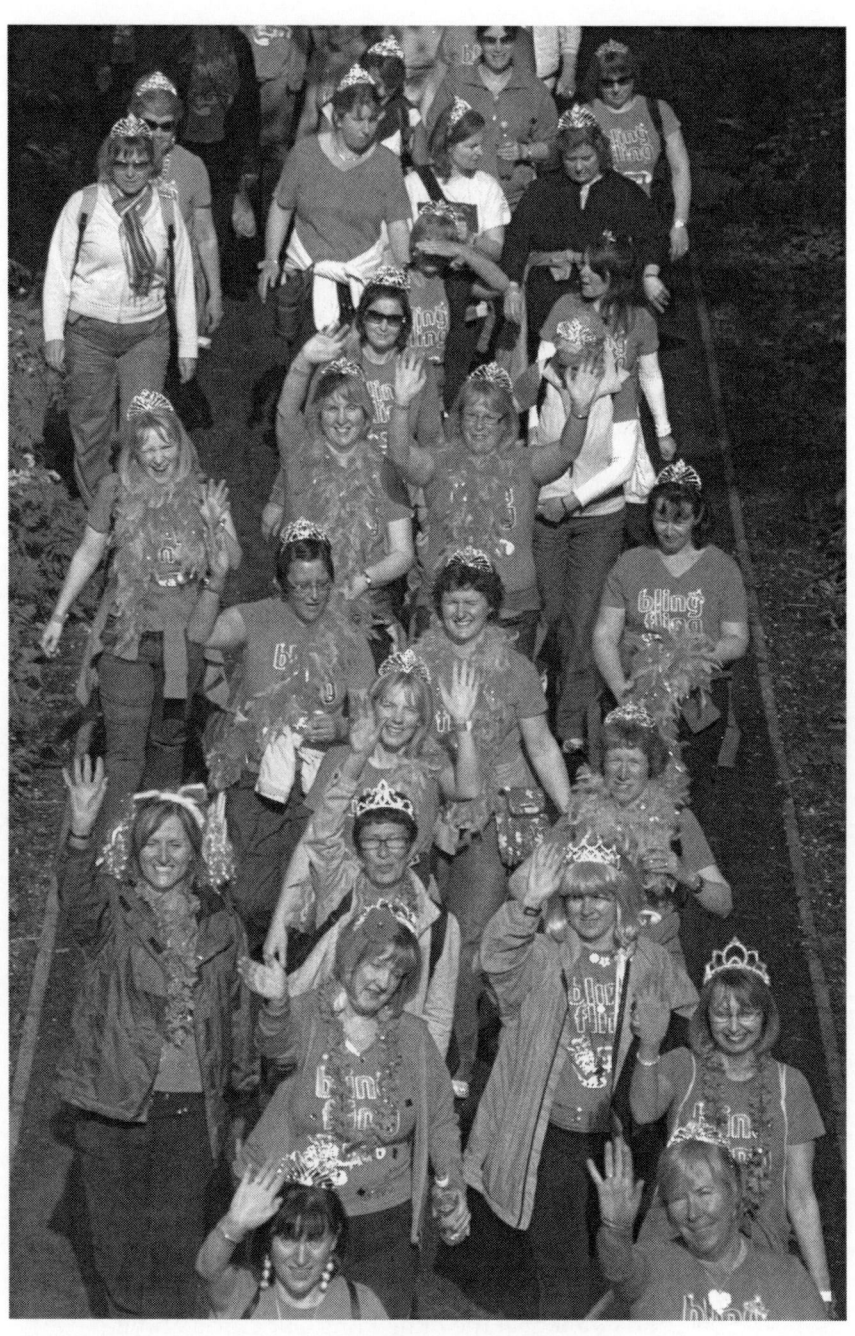

A sea of pink at the Bling Fling

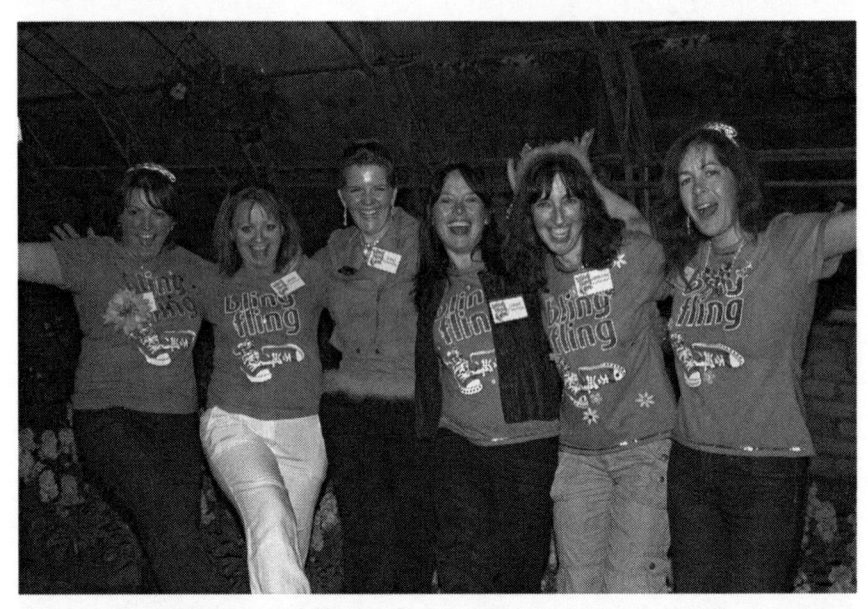

Doing It With Bling On - the girls from the committee

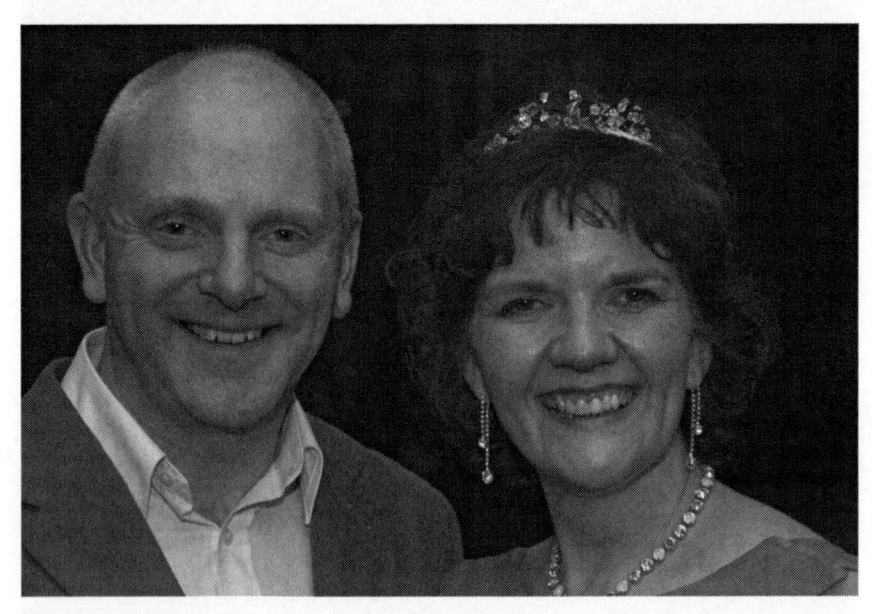

Sonja and Graham at the Bling Fling Christmas Thing

## Chapter 19

The day I got that new wig was marked with sadness. For that afternoon, just before my appointment, I went to the funeral of a young man from Gang Show, whom I had known from his childhood days.

He had joined the Gang as a Cub, I had directed him as a Scout and then Venture Scout, and finally, at the young age of 23, having travelled the world enjoying many adventures in Scouting, he had died in tragic circumstances.

Sitting through that service, with new wig on and the remnants of the chemotherapy drugs still coursing through my veins, I watched the impact of this young man's death on his friends and family.

The fragile line we cross between life and death was never more poignant to me than on that cold January afternoon. Here was I, and those around me in the medical world, battling to beat the breast cancer inside me… while we sat mourning grappling with the sense in this tragic and unnecessary waste of a young life…

In that moment, my resolve was renewed. My fight wasn't easy but it would be won, and whatever happened, I would never give up. Life is too precious to let it go without a battle.

**Yuk, you should see the stuff that just came out of my feet. That's Aqua Detox for you…. Sonja**

With the end of chemotherapy came another treat, courtesy of Clan House – the miracle foot bath that is Aqua Detox.

I was told that the sessions would involve me sitting with my feet in a basin of water, letting the Detoxification process cleanse me, ridding my body of the toxins left by the drugs. In the process, it would also improve my circulation and oxygenate my blood, resulting in an overall boost of my immune system. Not a bad result, I figured....

I would need six weekly sessions, to match the six sessions of chemotherapy administered over the last three months, and before each I would get a mug of peppermint tea served with a smile and some chat from the ladies at Clan.

Actually, that's not quite how it was advertised, but it was exactly how it happened, and the tea and chat alone was enough to have me signing up for the whole course. Quite how these toxins would be washed out through my feet is beyond me – in fact, it is still beyond me (even with the benefit of hindsight) – but it did seem to work, and anything that gets me to sit in one place for an hour has got to be a good thing.

And so it was that I ended up, trousers rolled up round my knees, feet in a glorified basin in true Ma Broon style, electrodes installed to attract the toxins, and chatting to the therapist Marie for an hour as the detox worked its magic. I say 'chat' because that was a big part of the experience for me. Marie is a terrific listener, and is also Clan's relaxation guru, specialising in meditation and healing techniques, which I always find intriguing, being the kind of person whose mind is always in overdrive and who struggles to shut off from the world.

Some weeks she taught me how to relax my thoughts, leading me through a healing session while my feet were stewing. Sometimes she taught me how to meditate, other days we just talked. And each time, residue left in the basin became less and less orange as the toxins were gradually flushed out through the soles of my feet. Strange but true … one of these things that I will never understand the science of – or even attempt to – but the sight of the toxins departing, after months of enduring them being injected in there, certainly gave this girl a boost.

After those first six sessions, the Aqua Detox continued monthly, and will end only when I no longer feel the need to go. Nowadays, the only toxins showing in the water afterwards are from the wine, coffee or chocolate consumed in the days before. The visible evidence of the benefits of a detox diet I guess...

**Had mammogram today. Tumour has shrunk to nothing! They couldn't find it. Hurrah! Will still see surgeon next week but all is good!**
**Sonja**

Oh yes... the best news in the world awaited me in the ultrasound department three weeks after chemotherapy ended.

Although the radiographer had a terrible cold, and I hadn't quite got used to staying around people who were obviously harbouring bugs without covering my face with a scarf in a strange pop-star-hiding-from-the-paparazzi-type fashion, I bravely laid myself out on the examination table while she glided the camera over my breast – yet again. You see? I told you my topless torso had been photographed more than a Page 3 model's...

She looked strangely at me before saying: "Can you remember where the lump was?" I pointed to the area, which she scanned again – still nothing.

Okay, let's go back to the original pictures – the ones taken at the Albyn Hospital at the first night. Even the scans from the mid-point check were rendered worthless, the tumour having been reduced so much by the previous three chemotherapy doses.

A studied look at the original scans later, she returned and went straight to the place of the tumour – or at least, where it was. The faintest shadow revealed all she needed to know. The tumour was gone, the chemotherapy had worked, and I was well on my way to battling back from breast cancer. That day, there was dancing in the streets of my celebrating heart...

**Hi Sonja, just got your message. Fantastic news. Can't wait to see you and share that celebration drink together.**
**- Sharon, friend in Australia**

**Great news. You are going to beat this! Mine's a double!!**
**Gordon Somers (Gang Show Stage Crew)**

# Breast Cancer Care Nurse

**Val Bain has been a Breast Cancer Care Nurse at Aberdeen Royal Infirmary for 12 years.**

Her advice to me throughout my journey made the most sense to me at the time, and enabled me to follow the route that best suited me through the breast cancer maze. I know others will do it differently, and so I had a chat with Val to find out how she sees the cancer journey. Here is her advice. I hope it is useful:

"The way to get through cancer treatment is by taking one step at a time. Don't look too far ahead, deal with each treatment as it comes along, and be who you are, stay true to yourself. Everyone will do it differently – there is not a right or wrong way to deal with it. If someone is a quiet or not a positive type of person, they are not going to change just because they have breast cancer. It is important that I work with that knowledge and encourage people to do it in their way.

For Sonja, it was important to keep normality in her life. It's good to have something to look forward and so, when Sonja suggested going to London, I could see it was important to her to make that journey, even though she was coming up for her second chemotherapy session. I suggested to her that if she felt up to it, to go for it – she did and had a wonderful time. It is important that ladies, as much as is possible, keep normality in their lives and do what they feel able to – these experiences make the journey through treatment a little easier.

Following a diagnosis of breast cancer, ladies say that what is important to them in their lives changes, as do their priorities. A diagnosis of breast cancer may change you but it can be a positive experience. For Sonja her family and friends were always important to her, but following her diagnosis, they became even more so.

"When I first met Sonja, I quickly realised she was a strong, capable person but vulnerable at the same time. She had her sister with her the first day we met and together they were facing the challenges of the afternoon in which she was seeing the oncologist for the first time. As professionals, I think we should remember that when people are facing such a huge challenge is it important that they are treated compassionately and that we listen to their needs in a sensitive way.

Starting out on your first chemotherapy session is a giant step into the unknown – not knowing what to expect or how you will feel afterwards. Nothing is more terrifying than the unknown and trying to anticipate how things will be as you embark on uncharted territory. If your first treatment is not a good experience it raises anxieties that you will feel poorly throughout the course of treatment. Sonja faced all her treatment – chemotherapy, surgery and radiotherapy with style and bling (as she would). I never saw her at the hospital without her lippie and looking a million dollars.

It was good to meet with Sonja and her sister. Sonja has a wonderful support network around in her family and friends. It is not one person who goes through a diagnosis of cancer and it can be just as difficult to the 'others' who want to help and support but are not sure how. The significant others in a breast cancer diagnosis often have a feeling of helplessness. I am sure there were times that Sonja's friends and family felt like this but they managed to be an inspiration to her as she was to them. They kept as much normality in her life as was possible but at the same time provided a listening ear and a shoulder to cry on. Sadly, not all ladies have this support network and as a breast care nurse I try to assess very quickly what support ladies have and work with this accordingly.

Like many women going through breast cancer treatment, Sonja has children and she decided to include them in her journey. Some ladies choose not to tell their children but children are perceptive and pick up that there is something wrong and the not knowing can be worse for them. Sonja used our children's books which help parents to explain breast cancer and treatments in a language that they understand. I advise ladies to be honest with their children but each mother knows her children best and it has to be her decision as to how she deals with this.

When it comes to the end of the treatment, 'others' see this as being the end... There may be a new hairstyle and regular visits to the hospital will have stopped. However, for many ladies the start of a new chapter in their lives is just beginning. What 'others' do not see is the impact a breast cancer diagnosis and treatments can have, they do not see the changes to the head and heart. To 'others' it's 'Oh that's brilliant, let's open the champagne. That's it over!" But it's not... it's actually just the beginning of learning to live with a breast cancer diagnosis."

Val has always been supportive of both my personal journey and the Bling Fling idea. On the day itself, she walked the 10km and afterwards, advised party goers on Breast Awareness.

She says "When Sonja started speaking about organising the Bling Fling, I wasn't surprised, having got to know her over the months. She is a dynamic type of person, and I knew she would throw herself into whatever she did. What I was surprised at is the amount of work that went into organising the Bling Fling. I was concerned that she was taking on too much just after finishing treatment, but once again her friends were there looking after her and making sure she did not take on too much.

I absolutely loved the day, it was such a fun time and wonderful to see so many ladies supporting the Bling Fling. Apart from substantial money raised for Prof Heys Breast Cancer Research, one of the things that came out of the Bling Fling was Sonja's friendships with all of the girls involved. It was an amazing testament to Sonja's journey and her ability to find a positive outcome in her situation."

# Chapter 20

E-mail to friend Sarah –

    **Date for your diary... I'm organising a walk (along with Lesley, Lisa, Pam, Lorraine and Janine) called the Bling Fling, with money being shared between Breast Cancer Research in Aberdeen, redecorating Ward 15 (chemotherapy day ward) and Archway.**
    **The theme for the night is Tiaras and Trainers!**
    **We're going to walk from Duthie Park to Cults and back, and will enjoy a Ladies Night with manicures, massages and music at the Winter Gardens when we return.**
    **It's on Sunday 17th May, starting at 5pm, and would be fab if you (and any girls you can muster?) could join us.**
    **Any potential sponsors wouldn't go amiss too!**
    **Sonja X**

The after effects of my final chemotherapy session probably lasted as long as the five others, but I was so busy by that time that I barely noticed. My heart was celebrating, the worst was behind me, and I had a new iron in the fire... and a need to strike while that iron was blazingly and piercingly hot.

With the Bling Fling idea firmly embedded and already taking root in my ever active imagination, I called a meeting of six friends who rushed in to join me, thinking about the consequences afterwards. I say consequences because I doubt that any of my talented and obliging pals ever had any idea what they were signing up for in the name of our friendship – they, like me, totally underestimated the hours, energy and creativity that would be spent on dreaming up the Bling Fling.

As it happens, we never expected to gain as much from the experience either... friendships were cemented, memories were shared and the sense of achievement was far greater than we would ever have imagined, making the whole Bling Fling project almost as life-changing for my friends as my breast cancer battle has been for me.

I chose six of the many, many people who have surrounded me over the last year. I have often had those e-mails – I have even forwarded them on occasion – asking me to choose six women who could work together and change the world, but this is the first time I had to put it into practise. What we achieved together has not exactly changed the world, granted, but it has changed many lives, including our own, and the money raised by the Bling Fling walkers will continue to change and save lives for many years to come.

I always knew that as well as having great friends, I was also surrounded by very talented women, all of them fantastic wives and mothers, whose other skills had been hidden from the world through their child-raising years. I recognised these friends had a range of different and contrasting skills to my own, skills that I have always admired and found fascinating, but have never known the depth of until we started working together on the Bling Fling.

The first person to join the Bling ranks was, of course, Janine. As co-conspirator and dream maker, she was the obvious choice to share the chairman duties – to be honest, I have always seen myself as more of a figurehead (not quite as wooden as that on the Cutty Sark, but certainly a pretty face with a penchant for talking a good line and winning people over) while Janine was the true backbone behind the committee, her history of fundraising for various charities in Aberdeen proving invaluable while setting out on this quest.

Janine knew how important it was for me to choose the other committee members, given the fact that the project was my baby in the first place, and she advised me to choose a few friends with varying skills, letting me loose to dream up the perfect team at breakneck speed. With only four months to play with, we had to work quickly - just as well decision-making is my forte and certain of my friends sprang to mind instantly as being potential partners in Bling.

With Janine and I already on board, we had the event organisation, marketing and fundraising expertise covered. Next we needed someone who had a head for figures – and Lesley, who had worked as a business manager before having her three lovely children, and having recently resigned from her post as treasurer to the PTA, seemed like the perfect choice. She is also, as I have already said, possessor of an amazing ability to laugh and what's more, make others laugh, which I knew would be the perfect antidote to boring committee meetings.

Having sat on several committees, I have to say I am not a fan of board membership – or should that be 'bored' membership? - and if this Bling Fling one was going to work, it had to be fun all the way, or I would lose interest before it had even started. Laughter, therefore, was completely necessary and supplied in bucketloads by Queen of Celebrity chat herself, Lady Lesley 'Frixinet'.

Les worked tirelessly over the next few months, creating Just Giving Accounts, bank accounts, setting up spreadsheets and logging the comings and goings of the fundraising efforts, which at the last count has seen the guts of £80,000 through its books in the first year. Her dining table has become an accountant's desk, her evenings a blur of calculators and income and expenditure columns, while as a committee we looked on in awe as we realised what Lesley was truly capable of....

Next we needed a list maker and an organised mind – two attributes to which my own scatty personality bears little witness, but skills which the Bling Fling most definitely needed in order to take root. Footing the bill in these areas was my neighbour Lisa, who with two little girls, one with autism, and a full and happy life which includes growing her own fruit and vegetables, baking wheat free muffins to die for (and if you've ever tried cooking wheat free anything, you'll know what a feat that is) as well as being a partner in her husband's business with years of experience in hotel management behind her, I knew she would be the very person.

The fact that she also wanted to try her hand at setting up websites and internet mailing systems – just for her own interest – and had many friends in the Aberdeen business world whom she could persuade to walk the Bling Fling or help with sponsorship was the icing on the cake... Once again, Lisa was the perfect choice. Lots of laughs, perfectly dependable and loyal to the end, she would also prove her abilities to us – and to herself - over and over again over the following months.

Organising an event like the Bling Fling is a massive task, and the hazards of such took on gargantuan proportions in the months running up to May. As I stood with my friend Pam in the playground watching a workman on the roof of a six-storey tenement clambering about without safety harness, while Pam turned green with the thought of what might happen, I knew she was the one to take on the mantle of keeping everyone safe.

Pam had until recently been PTA chairman, and had carried out the task so perfectly that no one wanted to follow her into the role. She had also worked as Project Manager in the Oil Industry and the NHS, had a history in Human Resources and is the kind of person who organises you without you even knowing you're being organised. She is another doer, a list-maker, an event organiser and a girl who likes to have fun – the fifth perfect choice for my merry band of Pink Sparkly Ladies.

Lastly there was Lorraine, who works as a Sister at the Children's Hospital and provided our necessary link with the National Health Service and an inroad into all its politics and quirky regulations. Although Lorraine holds down a full time job, as well as bringing up two beautiful daughters and icing cakes for anyone lucky enough to know of her domestic goddess skills, she pledged to help us as and when she could.

There was an ulterior motive for Lorraine's interest. Two of her colleagues had been diagnosed with breast cancer around the same time as I was, and as an extraordinary listener and adviser, Lorraine found herself being a friend and confidante to all three of us over the following months. Sadly, we couldn't all look forward to the same outcome, as you will discover, but for each of us, Lorraine was the common link which helped us find our journey to whichever destination we were headed.

In the end, when we raised more money than we ever thought possible, the children's hospital also gained from our efforts, with Bling Fling money being used to buy two chemotherapy chairs and a heart monitor for Lorraine's own day ward. Money from the follow-up Bling Fling Christmas Thing was given to the Children's Hospital to buy entertainment systems for children enduring long stays in hospital.

And so our small but perfectly formed committee was complete. No one was more surprised than I when, when I asked to help, my friends jumped in once more to fight my latest and entirely different cause ... one that would demand far more of them than just their time.

Our first meeting took place in January, over coffee, cakes and excited chatter in the comfortable surroundings of my living room, where the idea was bought and sold, planned and honed, formed and grown to become the sea of pink which would flood the old railway line in May that year.

At our weekly gatherings, the t-shirts were born, websites designed and implemented, press releases written and rewritten, logos mulled over the printed, participants registered, pink fizz tasted and chosen, food planned and organised, entertainment put in place and approved, all carried out by our small industrious committee as we felt our way through the charity walk minefield, each of us fulfilling roles and completing tasks that we had never before imagined ourselves capable of.

While our friendships grew stronger, the plans took shape, and within six weeks, we were ready to launch the Bling Fling Tiaras and Trainers walk idea on the Aberdeen public.... the middle of February date coinciding exactly with step two of my own personal battle which was still ongoing... operation D-day was upon me before I really had time to think...

    Check out the Bling Fling Website on www.blingfling.org and register to come and help me raise loads of cash for breast cancer research at ARI, Ward 15 Anchor Unit and Archway. Hope you can make it!

    **Good job on the website – looks fab. Erica X**

    **I'll be there. Think what you're doing is fab. Just don't want to miss it. Lots of love Fiona X**

## Message from my best and oldest friend Fiona

**Fiona made the journey from London to join me for the Bling Fling – six months from the day I travelled to London to join her birthday celebrations. This was her message:**

I am entering the Bling Fling because Sonja Read is a dear friend – my oldest friend – and I would not want to miss sharing this experience with her.

She has been remarkably brave and positive through her diagnosis and treatment of Breast Cancer – truly an inspiration - and I am very proud that my friend has gone one step further than most would to organise this event which will make a difference to all those who are treated with chemotherapy in Aberdeen.

I would like to add that I am not at all surprised that Sonja is doing all this as it is typical of her to be pretty amazing!

I am participating in the walk because I love Sonja and want to help to make the day a great success as I know it will be. I have friends and family whose lives have been affected by cancer and I am doing it for them too.

## Message to the Bling Fling Website from University friend Susan

Sonja is a great friend. We have known each other for over 20 years and she was the first to know when I got pregnant with my daughter Ailsa 16 years ago.

Sonja is an amazing person who has tackled her cancer treatment with her own inimitable style. How anyone can continue to look glamorous and stress-free amazes me.

I admire the effort and meticulous planning that the whole Bling Fling team are putting into this fabulous event.

Well done ladies. You are really demonstrating very powerfully what incredible things women can do when they pull together.

# Chapter 21

**All set? I will be thinking about you. Ailsa**

I'm not sure how 'set' I was for my hospital visit … although I had had good news all the way as far as chemotherapy goes, and I knew the tumour was no longer visible to the human eye, there was still doubt somewhere in the back of my mind that it wouldn't be the same story once I was under the knife.

The plan was to do a lumpectomy, removing any tissue damaged by the cancer, along with a few lymph nodes, to be checked for signs of cells having spread into my lymphatic system (and therefore, giving them the means to travel elsewhere in my body).

Although Professor Heys had told me time and time again that I had had the best possible response to chemotherapy, and this operation would have minimal impact, there was still that nagging fear that all would not look so rosy when he looked more closely, which I suppose is only natural given the circumstances.

As usual, however, I buried my worries by doing something I had some control over – I went shopping for the most glamorous pyjamas the hospital had ever seen. At least I would cut a dash around the ward, even though I was worrying myself sick inside at the thought of what was to come.

> **Morning babe. Hope you're feeling fine and good luck for today's operation. Another wee step on the way to recovery. Skerry X**

I had to check into hospital the day before my op – actually, I could have gone in early morning on the day itself, as long as I ate nothing from 8pm the night before (sounds rather like my instructions from the vet when my Persian cat goes in for his annual comb-out). But as all mums will appreciate, I fancied the rest that a night in hospital would bring. If I stayed home, I'd end up looking out school uniforms, making packed lunches, brushing hair, sorting out squabbles... you know the kind of thing. Every family has mornings like that, especially when mum has to be somewhere at a particular time.

So I checked myself in the night before, purely by choice, for a bit of rest and recuperation courtesy of the National Health Service. And how glad I am that I did.... because we had fun in that female surgical ward. Little sleep was had, but LOTS and LOTS of chat was to be found there...

> **Thanks for making my hospital stay fly by. It was quite a laugh! Lorraine**

Just before Christmas, and nearing the end of chemotherapy, I had been on a night out with the girls (I say girls, but perhaps ladies is more of an accurate description), from my adult tap class. We no longer dance together, more is the pity, but we still enjoy the social side that our classes fulfilled, getting together twice a year for a meal and catch up. You know the kind of thing that we women are exceptionally good at....

Anyway, that Christmas, a tap dancing friend of mine, Lorraine, had just been diagnosed with breast cancer. Her treatment was different from mine – no chemotherapy, straight on to the operation followed by a course of radiotherapy. So we knew we'd be going through our treatment around the same time.

It was still a surprise, however, to find her in the very next bed to mine – a veritable roommate at the hospital. What's more, Lorraine followed me into the scanning room on the morning of the operation, and I followed her into the operating theatre in the afternoon. We were there for each other as we slid gracefully under the effects of the pre-med, and again as we groggily recovered from the anaesthetic later that evening.

She shared the fruit her husband had brought in at visiting time (actually she told me later, it was her daughter who encouraged that particular purchase. Her husband, like mine, would never think of such a thing), and we chose huge plates of stovies from the hospital menu together, to be eaten on our last day before returning home. We laughed recently at the memory of phoning our husbands from the ward to stall them collecting us until after lunch, only so we could finish and enjoy the aforementioned Scottish delicacy.

I think without Lorraine and our hours of merry chatter, our hospital stay would have been a far less positive experience – thank goodness for friends and small worlds….

> **Lorraine, Yes, hospital was a laugh – most of it anyway! Great we went through it together. Can't think of a better roomie! Sonja X**

The constantly high temperature of the hospital ward forced me into doing something that until then I had managed to fight the urge – I went topless….

Before you fall of your chair at that shock revelation – or at the very least choke on your cuppa – what I mean is, I shed my wig and showed the world, or the medical world in which I was ensconced for the time being, my baldness.

As I stripped off in the relative privacy of the communal toilet, and headed out into the ward, shyly revealing the secret me to my ward mates – one of whom was also modelling the glorious results of chemotherapy drugs - no one batted a hairless eyelid. Lorraine said I was 'Lucky!' Huh? Lucky? 'To have such a lovely shaped head – I really suited my new look,' she added.

Within minutes I felt perfectly at home with my baby smooth bonce – even the cold wasn't a problem, despite the February snow falling outside. In that little ward, with my roommates around me, all going through various stages of breast cancer treatment, I did feel lucky. To have got that far. To still be smiling. And yes, especially to be the proud owner of a lovely round head.

I did have one regret about going commando, however... which came when I forgot to put my wig back on for a visit to the out patients' for a mammogram. Of course, me being me, and Aberdeen being Aberdeen, I came face to face with a very glamorous, very beautiful lady that I've known for years but seldom see, and suddenly felt exposed and vulnerable without my crowning glory. I'm sure if I hadn't spoken, she would never have recognised me – strangely, people find it hard to recognise a face when it's not adorned with its usual style or colour of hair. Many old friends have walked past me in the last few months – even when my own hair had started re emerging at the end of chemotherapy – and not known who I was until I opened my big mouth and sounded forth with the latest gossip or my own inimitable laugh.... inherited from my dear dad and embarrassingly recognisable in crowds.

The other lesson I learned from my topless in public episode is that I had been right to opt for the anonymity of wig-wearing. I drew this conclusion when sitting in the waiting room, next to a lady who told me she was accompanying her daughter for a mammogram. Obviously worried about the findings, and panicking she may be about to follow me down a road I was so obviously marching before her, she poured out all her fears and anxieties as I listened, wishing I had not labelled myself in such an obvious manner.

Don't get me wrong, I usually love a good natter with a stranger, and am quite at home with making small talk. I'll even find joy in cheering others up when they are experiencing their own difficult time, but at that point in my life, I was not ready to burden myself with other people's cancer stories or fears. Now that I am through the worst, I can take whatever is thrown at me, but just at that moment, I was being selfish, keeping my own bald but carefully covered head above water, so that I could keep my worries under my wig and project an aura of confidence and high spirits to the world around me.

**Hi there. Just to let you know I'm thinking of you!**
**Good luck and see you soon, Catriona X**

Just as Lorraine and I tuned in to the chat and daytime television that a stay in hospital can bring, Prof Heys and the anaesthetist provided the welcoming party to herald the events of the next 24 hours – the real reason we were here as it were... just in case we had any illusion it was all going to be fun.

Actually, there is lots of fun to be had with the Prof around, and with an anaesthetist promising to massage my hand as I went off to sleep and then provide acupuncture throughout my operation, I was already beginning to believe my self-induced illusion that I had entered a health farm and could chill out for the next few days. Not a bad impression to have when trying to forget about the real task in hand, and in fact, the perfect dream to escape to when hearing about lymph nodes and lumps about to be removed from my 40-year-old body while I enjoyed the deepest most relaxing sleep I had had for some time.

> **Hi Soggers. Good luck with the op today. Hope everything goes well. We're all thinking of you.
> Love Keith, Claire, Ev, Jojo and Flynnbo**

Now, remember the problem they'd had in locating my lump at a recent ultrasound test? Well, things didn't get much better the morning of the operation.

The ultrasound department had been given the task of marking the now invisible lump, which should have been quite an easy process, given the equipment and expertise at their disposal.

However, easy did not enter the vocabulary that morning, as I sat, tummy rumbling (I'd had no breakfast in preparation for the op remember) and had markers shoved into me from every angle. Actually, I say markers, and you'll probably imagine something small and insignificant. In fact, these markers were more like wires of the type I last saw in jewellery making workshops, shoved in and taped down so the end didn't poke me in the eye! That gives you an idea of the length and dangers of the task involved.

Anyway, each wire was administered with painstaking precision, followed by a mammogram to ascertain if they'd hit the spot.... and therein lay the problem.

For each time they positioned the needles, then had a look through the metal plates of the previously described and painfully remembered George Fornby grill sensory experience, they realised they were nowhere near the location in question – and went back to the drawing board to begin the whole complicated procedure again...

After the third attempt, the consultant decided just to do a 'belt and braces job on me' and placed in as many needles as he could, all converging on the spot where 'he suspected the lump might have been'. In the end, the Prof confided surreptitiously afterwards, not one of the needles in my pin cushion of a breast actually led to the cells in question, but the will had been there, and I was pleased not to be a run-of-the-mill textbook case.

The time spent on me meant Lorraine was kept waiting for her pre-op tests, time she spent wisely and well, entertaining the troops while in her dressing gown, and catching up on the latest copy of a celebrity magazine, tales with which she would regale me afterwards as we became sleepily and lovingly drunk on our pre-med tipple.

When she eventually was seen, incidentally – I was amused to hear they had injected blue dye into her breast tissue which would flow into her lymph nodes, thus guiding the Prof when he came to removing them... the thought of the lasting colour this dye would leave gave me no option but to rename Lorraine the Blue Tit for the remainder of our hospital stay....

Lorraine left for her op just as I was given my lovely lunchtime cocktail from the locked drug store. The last time I had enjoyed such a pleasant afternoon I had been on a ship sailing towards Barbados while sipping Pina Colada on the deck and catching a few rays as the children swam in the nearby pool. Then, I felt sleepy and in love with the world – and I have to say, this pre-med tranquiliser did quite the same with bells on.

I was carried away in a dreamlike trance, brought back to reality at one point by the nurse, who revealed some important information from Lorraine, who had gleaned some vital information she thought I'd like to know. 'Em, Sonja, sorry to wake you but Lorraine wants to know if you've got cotton pants on...'

'Huh? What? I'm drifting on the Carribbean sea here, cocktail in hand... who cares what kind of pants I've got on....'

'Only, she's just had to remove hers for the op... nylon mix creates static in the operating theatre. She just thought you'd like to know...!'

And so, I leapt to life for a few minutes to carry out the relatively unglamorous task of changing my pants to a cotton pair, to save my face on the operating table, when of course, I'd be out for the count and would remember nothing about my modesty anyway.... the things a girl will do in pursuit of glamour...

My trip from the ward to the operating theatre was like a scene from Casualty, a particular television favourite of my wee sister Erica who, no matter how busy her life, will always find time for an hour of highly believable accident scenarios A&E style. Hurtling through the hospital while lying in a drunken stupor on a cot bed is a surreal experience - you end up counting the lights, looking for cracks in the ceiling, struggling to keep tabs of the conversation going on around you. I've never had an out-of-body experience before, but I'm sure this must be what it feels like, looking down on yourself lying there in a loose fitting, leave-nothing-to-the-imagination hospital gown, while the hustle and bustle of the NHS goes on around you. Not quite connected, but right in the midst of everything. The last time I felt that way I think I was 18 and just about to head for the nearest toilet at a student party.... the next time the door came to a halt somewhere nearby.

When my little entourage finally reached our destination – the clinical cleanliness of the operating theatre, deep in the heart of the hospital – wig and pride abandoned somewhere along the way, I remember seeing the Prof and the anaesthetist, counting to three... and then nothing... I woke up a couple of hours later without so much as a hangover. Groggy with sleep, desperate for food and with a mouth like a badger's armpit, as we used to say in Student Show days after a particularly lively night out, but happy and not in the least bit worse for wear from the highly potent cocktail I'd enjoyed in lieu of lunch.

I had two huge plasters, one over the lump area and one under my armpit – plasters which I knew would be the envy of my daughter (who has always had a fascination for them, although this particular mummy very seldom administers them, not being a true believer in their healing abilities. If fresh air was good enough for me, it's good enough for my own tiny warriors...). But as far as I could tell, the Prof had done what he expected to do, the lump was gone, my breast was still there, and some lymph nodes had been removed for testing...

I was happy, and very very hungry, which called for one thing, and one thing only... some tea, toast and ward chat to celebrate.

Lorraine and I talked and laughed for hours that night – we had slept half the day, I suppose, and were being administered painkillers like sweets from the sweetie trolley, so catching some shuteye was never going to come easily, no matter how much relaxation therapy I put it into practise in the dim light of the ward.

I had also sent out a text before heading for Bedfordshire as they say, and my phone hardly stopped with replies...

> Hi – all went well! Bit sore but nothing a few days won't fix. Love Sonja X

> What a girl! One more bit done and dusted. Sleep well, Ailsa X

> Well done, been thinking about you. Take care. See you at home. Ian X

> I've been thinking of you. Glad it went well. Rest tonight and will catch up soon. Lisa X

> Hi, good to hear things went well. Sarah and I missed you at the Art opening tonight. Hope they have given you a good dose of valium? Sandy

> Great news. You have been brill. Look forward to seeing you. Lesley X

The morning after, I was back to normal - showering, doing my make-up, putting on my wig – all set to face the outside world with the positivity and style it had come to expect – and I had come to expect of myself.

When the Prof did his rounds that morning, both Lorraine and I were in high spirits, heightened by the news that everything had gone smoothly, he had removed seven nodes, he had managed to find the lump – or what was left of it – and he had already spent the morning teasing the consultant radiographer about his efforts to locate it.

The Prof's round was followed by the physiotherapist, who talked me through returning to exercise – starting with the beginners task of swinging my arm gently by my side daily, up to the grand challenge of raising it high above my head after three weeks. The fact that I could do the final task just twelve hours after surgery, and was already making plans to return to choreographing the Gang Show a few days later may have seemed reckless to her... but as she didn't seem too perturbed by my plan, I went off again to listen to my body and do what I felt capable of .... my tried-and-tested method which had worked for me throughout breast cancer treatment, was put into practise yet again.

With all the peptalks done, paperwork sorted out and drugs administered – enough paracetemol to last me through the next two years of colds and period pain (which did return over the following months) – all that remained for Lorraine and I to do was to enjoy our last supper of stovies together before heading out into the winter wonderland of a snow-dusted February day.

Graham came to collect me half an hour before the children were due to come out of school, and although I'd arranged for a friend to bring them home where I would be waiting, I felt so well that I decided to go to the playground myself.

As Matthew and Emma emerged, they clocked me, and faces beaming with surprise and delight, started running, both smiling fit to burst and teary with relief. As they collided in front of me, flinging their arms around my waist, I buried my head in their baby-soft hair, smelled their familiar smell and cherished that moment. As I emerged from the embrace and looked around, I realised that every mummy in the playground that afternoon was watching us, eyes filled with tears... anyone who has ever known the love of a child, will appreciate the emotional journey of that snow-filled day.

**Doing fine – glad to be home. Lots of love Sonja X**

# Matthew's Story

**My son Matthew was ten when I was diagnosed. He remembers his shock and how the reality wasn't quite as bad as he imagined at the outset...**

Finding out mum had breast cancer was sudden for me because I had absolutely no idea that that she would come home from hospital that day and say she had cancer. It was a big shock.

I remember feeling angry when mum told us her hair was going to fall out because I was worried I was going to be embarrassed and I thought my friends might tease me about my mum being bald. But everything turned out okay in the end. I didn't have anything to worry about.

When we were choosing the wig with mum it was pretty hard because she kept saying no to the ones we liked. The most important thing to me was that mum looked the same.

The day that dad shaved mum's head, Emma and I were hiding underneath the bedcovers in their room because it was a bit frightening and I knew mum was upset. I suppose it was pretty funny in a way – mum looked a bit strange when she was bald, but I got used to it. Then she changed her wig, which I had to get used to again.

Mum had lots of changes over those months and we got used to all of them. I didn't get used to her being bald though because she never really was, except when she was sleeping. Mum and dad were two baldies in bed. I didn't want to see mum's head – and I'm glad she wore her wig all the time. I always had a vision of what mum would look like bald but she didn't look anything like that.

When mum got her hair cut the weekend before she started wearing her wig, everyone said she looked like me, which was pretty embarrassing. I didn't think she was nearly as handsome as I am!

When her hair started to grow back in at the end it was okay because it grew quickly and it didn't take long before she looked okay again. None of my friends said anything about it – I didn't get made fun of at all. I think mum coped pretty well and she always looked pretty good. I was proud of her.

The first person I told that mum had breast cancer was my teacher. She helped by cheering me up. She read me the book that I'd brought in, and a few of my friends gathered round when she was reading. It was nice of her to do that. It helped me a lot.

I tried to keep it a secret from most people and it sort of worked. I thought if I told them they'd make fun of mum and that would make me upset. I don't know what I thought they would say, but they never really did say anything about it.

I never thought mum would die of cancer because this is a modern day and age and I didn't really think it would be a problem because all the doctors know what they are doing.

I really enjoyed going to the CLAN Children's Group. They gave us great opportunities to do fun things that we'd never done before – like a trip round Pittodrie, Aberdeen's Football Stadium. It was fun and I enjoyed it.

It was nice to meet other children there too. I've never asked about anyone, but people have told me about their mum or dad who had cancer. I think we could speak to each other because it's like speaking to a friend, to someone we could trust and someone who knows what you mean because they have been through this too.

I don't think anything really bad happened the year mum had breast cancer. There was nothing particularly wrong with it – everything went well. My best memory was mum getting her head shaved – that was pretty funny! I also liked having a sleepover on a school night, which we did when mum went into hospital for her operation.

When mum came out of hospital we were very happy. I saw her waiting in the playground and I was excited and so pleased to see her there looking just the same.

Mum was the same all the way through her breast cancer treatment, and everything was pretty normal most of the time. I think she did well to do it like she did and I'm very proud of her.

# Chapter 22

**Hi Sonja, Just thinking about two weeks ago and wondered how you were. I'm fine – no word from hospital yet but guess that's normal. Hope you are fine and taking it as easy as you can ... Lorraine X**
**Feeling fine. Still a bit tired and sore and itchy at times – but I guess it's just healing. Not driving yet but otherwise good, Sonja X**

As roommates in the hospital ward, Lorraine and I had supported one another, laughed and cried together, eaten stovies together and now were partners in recovery. In those first few weeks, we texted and spoke regularly, comparing notes and talking one another through treatment yet to come.

Now, many months down the line, Lorraine and I still meet for a chat, and even when out in a crowd with our fellow dancers, we end up laughing at memories of those couple of days spent together at ARI. Not one of those memories is sad or emotive either, which goes to show just why it is so important to find the fun in a situation, however hard to find that fun it may be.

Confined to Shanks' Pony when I first emerged from hospital, or depending on friends to drive me around, I felt I had found my vocation in life.... If I'm honest, I have always fancied myself as something of a Lady Penelope, so being chauffeur-driven around town suited my bling-and-growing-blingier-by-the-minute image.

I also did lots of walking, and as the winter passed and Spring beckoned, my friends and I found ourselves out on the Old Deeside Railway Line yet again, cycling, walking and planning the route for the Bling Fling which was now well on the way to launch date....

**Taking paper stitches off today so all good – feeling fine! Sonja X**

Everyday skills like showering were soon mastered, as I became accomplished at washing my wounds with my back to the jet, keeping my plasters dry as instructed and then patting and rubbing in Aqueous Cream to aid healing. Not only have I been left eight months later with a barely visible wound – in fact, the Prof recently observed that if you didn't know I'd had breast surgery, you wouldn't know and as such, I was a great advert for his handiwork. My skin also sailed through the weeks of radiotherapy to come, whether or not as a result of the layers of moisture built up over those weeks of cream rubbing and massage, I'll never know, but at least it made me feel I had some say over the outcome, control freak that I had become.

As I recovered, Gang Show week drew closer, providing me with another new focus as I found myself running towards the next self-imposed finishing line finding the laughs on the way. Pulling out the stops in the run up to the show, I lost myself somewhere between rehearsals and costume checks, band calls and staging meetings as the show came together and, in spite of everything being stacked against its success due to my diagnosis at the beginning of rehearsals, it was once again declared 'Aberdeen's best Gang Show yet...'. Maybe something to do with the fact that I had done more delegating than usual. Note to self for future reference – delegate more, do less. Others can do it just as well as you, and will benefit from the chance to try.

This year has taught me some valuable lessons, and not trying to be all things to all people is one of them. Be true to yourself, listen to your head and enjoy everything you do. The world will go on revolving without you, but it's more fun to keep well enough to stick around for the ride....

The week of the show was fun in so many ways, but in others it brought home to me the journey I had come so far. I met many people I knew during Gang Show week – as I always do, having been around it for over 20 years - and I had to go through my story so often that I ended up avoiding the audience if I could, sticking by my production team friends who had travelled some of the journey with me and didn't have to be talked through every step along the way. That way I could enjoy myself, laugh lots, feel the same as I always felt during show week and stay firmly 'on my perch', which by that time would have been easily pushed from underneath me. The volcano of my emotions was just about to blow. I'd held onto my positivity for as long as I could, and any day now, the framework that I had built around me was about to shatter.

For now, however, I lived in the moment, enjoyed the ride, got sad once or twice – mainly when watching the girls straightening or curling their hair (always a wrench when in mourning for my golden locks, which although growing in, weren't quite covering enough to save me from being labelled a 'cancer victim' if I went baldy, a label which I would avoid at all costs), or when people were singing my praises and thanking me for my efforts at the end of the week. To be honest, those heartfelt thankyous always prompt a tear but at this stage I was so vulnerable that as soon as anyone mentioned the battle I had undertaken to get that show on stage, the tears were never too far away.

**Doing fine today. Cycled out railway line and had coffee with friends ... great! – Text from Sonja**

**Karen passed your message onto the dance class last night. Glad to hear you're doing well. Look forward to seeing you soon Text from Lindsey, dance class friend**

Every day was different at that stage, and facing the challenges of one day at a time meant that my life was something of a rollercoaster for a while.
The good days found me with friends or the children, cycling, at dancing class, walking, having coffee, chatting, laughing and

planning the Bling Fling (which incidentally was my next finishing line).

Not so good days were filled with fear, sadness, mourning for my hair, for my health, for the life that I used to have and the worries I was yet to face...

When I woke each morning, I would never know which mood I would be in – often it depended on what I was doing that day. If I was busy and had lots to focus on, plenty of dates for my diary as it were, I would cope and often have a very happy day.

If I had a day to myself, I would sit and think and retreat into my cave where it was hard to see the light, never mind the finishing line.

The funny thing is, although I knew where the problems lay, I also knew I had to spend time alone with my thoughts. I needed to go through this mourning process – for myself, for my life as it was, for all those around me. I knew I had changed, I knew my outlook would and could never be the same again, and I knew I had to give myself the time and space to adjust to that mindset.

However hard it was, I also knew I would get there eventually...

**Hi honey, Just thinking of you and hoping you are okay. I know you were feeling a bit down. I think after everything you've been through and the energy you've put into being so positive, you maybe need to give yourself permission to feel down about it. Remember we are all here for you and if there is anything you need, just ask. Love Kay (Book group friend)**

By the time Ian and I went along to Clan the week after Gang Show ended, to hand over a cheque for £800 donated into collection buckets by our very generous audience, I had reached crisis point.

It took only a few kind words from the delighted fundraising manager there to set me off – and even as I cried, I was still joking, trying to make them believe I was alright, just being silly, emotional, a bad case of post-show blues. (Actually, I have suffered from post show blues before – when I was much younger and performing roles onstage, I would often mourn the passing of show week and spend at least a day in the deepest darkest depths of depression before focussing on the next one and starting the rehearsal process all over again, only to fall in love with my next role with an equal undying passion.) This time, however, was different, and as such, it needed careful handling.

Before I left Clan House that day, the fundraiser had encouraged me to sign up for a session with one of their specialist counsellors, a task I did indeed carry out eventually – but not for a couple more months. For the moment, I was not quite ready to accept that I needed help. As far as I was concerned, I was coping, I just needed time to get over Gang Show, to refocus on the Bling Fling, and to head off in the direction of another finishing line.

There was also good news heading my way, which would put the spring in my step to tide me over another few weeks...

**Tumour all gone ... Val called this morning to say they took a while to find it but all the tissue they took out is clear! Start radiotherapy after Easter! Sonja**

**So glad you got good news too. You deserve it! Lorraine**

You see? Good news WAS just around the corner – the tumour was gone, the wound was healing nicely and, the best news, we could have an Easter break before starting on six weeks of daily radiotherapy.

By that time, I can tell you, we all needed that holiday – and a week at Loch Tay with my old friend Linsay and her family was the perfect opportunity to rest and play together – and for me to launch yet another – and this time final - new look on the world.

**Bling Fling Website ready and registrations started... sign up and come and join us NOW!**

We first launched the Bling Fling website on Facebook, and as a forwarding e-mail around our personal address lists, requesting that friends send it to anyone they thought may be interested. Each of us pushed send... and then stood back and waited with slightly baited breath...would it work? And would it capture the imagination and go on working?

It seemed we'd hit the jackpot first time, when within minutes we were having hits on the freshly launched website, and within days the registrations were coming in... and they kept coming. In the end, over 400 women were willing to glam up in pink and bling and join us to raise cash for our very personal causes... and what's more, we were still turning people away right up to the big day itself.

Having spent 20 years writing for a local newspaper, I knew my colleagues at the Evening Express were keen to support my effort, and so as a committee we arranged a photograph to be taken at the Park, featuring us in evening dress and a stretch pink hummer, complete with chauffeur which was loaned to us for the evening – are you spotting a Lady Penelope theme here?

We seized the opportunity to have a girls' night in and plan our outfits for the modelling assignment. As well as a chance to chat – which we can never have enough of - it was also a reasonable excuse to try some of the pink fizz we were working our way through in preparation for the Bling Fling party. In fact, every time we got together over those couple of months, we seized the chance to try out yet another type of pink fizz. It's a hard job but somebody has to do it.... and as usual, we did it in style.

Once we were tanked up on friends, fun and fizz, we all decided we looked gorgeous in our outfits – don't we always through the bottom of a champagne glass? - chose tiaras to match (from our children's toy boxes) and got ready to party ..... on top of a hummer. And therein lies a funny story....

**To Bling Fling Girls – Pics being taken on Mon at 5.30pm at Duthie Park. Hope suits all? Sonja**

We turned up at the Duthie Park at the arranged time to find no photographer and a rapidly failing light. A few unanswered calls to the newspaper later – it was teatime after all, and journalists who work for the dailies make a sharp exit once the last edition has flown off the presses - someone finally ascertained that the photographer was waiting for us in another car park at the opposite end of the park. They would call her and send her over to meet us.

By the time we made contact, almost an hour had passed, and bearing in mind we were in full evening dress, even our jackets over our skinny straps failed to keep our teeth from chattering on that cool spring evening. We took refuge on the leopard skin seats of the Playboy hummer while we waited – and to give the evening yet more class, sang along to the in-built karaoke machine while sipping on more pink fizz...

When the photographer found her models, therefore, we were well on our way to partyville, with the wine going straight to our frozen brains without stopping at go.

When she then suggested I should sit on the bonnet of the car for the photograph, it seemed like a fun plan, and feeling invincible, I handed my glass to Pam and made my way up onto the very pink and very shiny vehicle like an intrepid mountaineer bagging her next Munro...

Note the fact the vehicle was very shiny ... my clothes were also very shiny, and together, they were so shiny that I slipped right off, pink fizz in hand, landing in a heap on the ground below as my friends looked down on me and laughed...

Not one 'How are you?' 'Oh no, she's got breast cancer, now she's fallen off a stretch hummer'.... zippo.... just lots and lots of laughter .... and a huge purple bruise to last me right up to the Bling Fling and beyond.

Actually bruising like a peach is another phrase that took on a whole new meaning after chemotherapy – my bruises were spectacular, shocking and instantaneous, and happened however sore the initial injury was. Matthew took great delight in pressing a finger to my leg and running off shouting 'Bruise...' A mean trick but it worked every time for months until my body had fully recovered from the chemotherapy drugs. My legs were a veritable rainbow of colour with many of the bruises having not so much as a story to explain their very existence.

But you know that fall went down in history as one of the best memories of our Bling Fling journey... it was hilarious, and I love having a story like that one to recount in a dull moment. As long as it is followed by a long, resounding laugh shared between friends, every bruise gained in the process was worth it.... and that one was truly spectacular.

Hey Gav, fell off the bonnet of a pink stretch hummer last night! You'd have loved it, Sonja

Is it on camera? Gav

No everyone too busy laughing to think about it! I had a glass of fizz in hand – didn't spill a drop! Pure class! Sonja

# Chapter 23

**Hi Sonja! We were wondering if you had anything planned for the Easter holiday? We are going to Kepranich at Loch Tay and if you would all like to join us for the April week, we would really enjoy your company. The children would love to have M & E to run around the field / play in the burns with....now they are older, if they have friends there, we just don't see them and they come back for food, the loo, or just to warm up. (They aren't allowed near the loch however, or the threat is you get grounded!) You can let me know if that suits.**

My friend Linsay is a true gem. Sensible and level-headed through and through, she is the ying to my yang... We shared a flat together in our years of singledom, and she inspired in me an interest in cookery, dress-making and home making that has never left me. I, in turn, bring my sparkle and sense of fun to our friendship. I can entice her to sit up late into the night, drinking wine and laughing, and I can persuade her to buy that new outfit that she doesn't really need but her life would be a whole lot brighter if it were hanging in her wardrobe.

Linsay is the kind of person who always makes you feel at home, she has a hot water bottle at the ready at bedtime, and a pair of slippers warming by the fire when you wake. Her husband Neil also knows how to keep a girl happy - with a bottle of wine always on hand (a skill he put to good use as one of our pink fizz volunteers at the Bling Fling) and an ever open offer to play football with the children, or take them out for a few hours so we mums can enjoy some girlie chat time or a catch up of our latest book group offering together.

Graham and I had been to Linsay and Neil's cottage at Loch Tay before and knew the healing benefits of Perthshire's gorgeous scenery and laid-back pace. We also knew that the children would have a ball catching up with Linsay and Neil's fun-packed pair, Alex and Brodie, and what's more, we all needed a holiday. With radiotherapy just around the corner, and months of worry now behind us, a week in Loch Tay was exactly the kind of holiday we had in mind.

And so, with bike rack in tow and the car boot packed full with wellies, waterproofs and all the warm clothes our wardrobes could muster, we set off on my pre-radiotherapy adventure which would provide the perfect venue for my 41$^{st}$ birthday celebration.

A year before, Erica had declared my 40$^{th}$ birthday 'more celebrated than Jesus Christ's' which of course was not strictly true but raised a laugh at the time... but truth be told, she was right in that I had indulged in a good few weeks of celebration.

The highlight of my 40$^{th}$ – apart from the aforementioned cruise – had been a day trip to Edinburgh, organised by Nicola, which took on something of the feel of my later chemotherapy sessions. She had asked each of my friends to bring something to add to the day – drinks, croissants, strawberries, chocolate, birthday cake, magazines – all to be read and consumed on the train journey down to our shopping trip, the highlight of which for me was a visit to the wonderful Vintage Shops which Auld Reekie has to offer.

When, a few months later, I was diagnosed with breast cancer, I focussed on getting through my battle by the time I reached 41, when I promised myself I would celebrate my 40$^{th}$ year all over again – because I was worth it.

Therefore, my 41$^{st}$ birthday took on far more importance than is usual for a 41-year-old, and my mid-life crisis turned into a mid-life rebirth, as I enjoyed the renewed zest for life that becoming a breast cancer survivor gave me.

Linsay and I had met up a few months before, when I took Emma on a pre-Christmas shopping day to Edinburgh, with the sole purpose of checking out Santa at Jenners. Of course, Santa being Santa and Jenners being Jenners, the old fella was booked up with visitors that particular Saturday, but Emma being my daughter declared she would rather have a manicure anyway, and ended up with snowflakes adorning her tiny nails which she showed off proudly as we passed the queue to the grotto which was growing ever longer.

That day, Emma and I met up with Linsay and her daughter Alex to take a wander round the lights, sounds and wonderful smells of the Christmas Festival in Princes Street Gardens. Looking the part of a Christmas elf, my red hair was covered with a Holly red hat and jacket which has been used on occasion as a Santa's Little Helper, and my old friend and I laughed and shivered together while warming our hands on steaming mugs of hot chocolate as the children took to the Helter Skelter, breathless with excitement and giggling with the carefree happiness of which childhood is made.

When we were invited to Loch Tay four months later, I was still wearing that red hat and jacket, but the sparkle that had been attributed to them over Christmas had faded in the winter months to follow. That Easter holiday, I followed my own lead of the October before and decided the time had come to launch my last new look on the world.

Where in October I had started wearing my wig in London, in April I went commando in Loch Tay - my hair short but there, an all-over covering which was dry before I had even left the shower, but it was mine, all mine, and I was ready to face the world again with my much admired high cheekbones and ever present dimples revealed for all to see.

Returning to the hairdresser for a quick tidy up before I bared my all was a scary prospect. Although I thought I looked alright, very few people – apart from the children and Graham – had seen the ravaged results of my chemotherapy hairdo, and I braced myself for Kirsteen's reaction once again.

This time, however, there were no tears or sadness as I removed my wig. Instead, she gasped in delight as she realised my hair was returning – curly, darker and very, very short, but returning, as thick and healthy as ever.

Loch Tay was the start of the sporty me ... the high cheekboned, tiny eared me with a smile to light up my face and eyes which seemed more prominent than before, only because they had no distractions and could work their magic as only eyes do... The windows to the soul revealed in full and glorious technicolour, and framed once more by a full set of fabulous eyelashes and eyebrows...

I remember so well the day I stopped wearing my wig. The children were at a holiday club in the local community centre, and I went to collect them, dressed in military style jacket, black and white striped scarf, usual bling brooch adorning my collar like a medal, and newly revealed, very short and stylish haircut.

Once more, there was a heart-warming moment as the children realised I was showing the world the me they had woken up to each morning, just before I assumed my disguise to face the rest of the day. Of course, the children, like Graham, had seen me in all my various stages of hair fall-out and regrowth – comfortable and stylish though wigs are, they still get tight and itchy after a day's wear and the relief of pulling on a woolly hat of an evening was comparable to stepping into a pair of your comfiest slippers after a day in stilettos.

Although the children were well aware of how I looked, they still appeared slightly shocked to see me waiting for them, minus wig, confidently sporting the boyish crop I had been hiding for weeks. They checked for my reaction... any shyness or under-confidence on my part would have instigated uncertainty on theirs. After a moment's pause, during which I could see them both searching my face for clues, they smiled, ran towards me and proudly showed me – and my new hairstyle – off to their friends.

To my – and I'm sure their – great relief, everyone approved – loved it even - and within seconds I was surrounded by a group of admirers, both children and adults, all asking the questions I have been answering ever since: 'Is that your natural colour?' (I don't know, I've been dying it for years!); 'Was it curly before?' (No, not unless I made a HUGE mistake with the heated rollers!); 'You've got no grey – you're so lucky!' Hmmm.... lucky? To lose my hair and have it come in again, dark and curly when it has been long and blonde all my adult life... well, I guess, lucky that there is no grey does put a positive spin on the whole rather traumatic experience.

Of course, the children's friends got a shock to see my hair quite so short. As I said, wearing a wig had led them all into an illusion that nothing was happening, and let me go through the battle in private with a sense of normality about my life. Revealing the results of chemotherapy exposed the truth to everyone, giving them a window on the journey I had so far travelled within the confines of my own family and closest friends.

By ditching my wig, I was letting everyone in – but by now I was able to cope with their reactions. I even loved their reaction to the latest me which was, without a doubt, the strongest and most striking image I'd ever had. Bright red lips, huge dangly ear rings, fabulous eye make-up designed to make my peepers seem bluer and deeper than ever before, and of course clothes – my waistcoats and pin-striped trousers taking on a whole new look when twinned with my no-nonsense hair and hairband, which I took to wearing in an attempt to bling up my new image... a girly twist to my boyish look as it were. Recently, one of the therapists at Clan said when she thinks of me she thinks of hairbands, and my rapidly growing collection has become something of a trademark look on my rapidly growing hair.

And so to Loch Tay, where Linsay, Neil and their children were waiting to entertain us, pamper us, cook for us, have lochside fires with us and cycle with us among some of the most stunning scenery Perthshire has to offer.

The sight of my short hair attracted the attention of Linsay's son, who at seven, found it hard to keep his thoughts to himself. His big sister on the other hand, had learned to think before she spoke – a trick that some adults have struggled to master.

The first time Brodie said 'You've got REALLY short hair', I could sense Matthew bristling defensively. I answered as I always did – 'Actually Brodie, I've got really long hair – you should have seen it a few months ago!' That cut his gas down to a peep for a few hours, until he got brave and curious yet again... 'WHY is your hair so short?' I answered, but being seven, he was still curious....

When he'd asked for the umpteenth time about my hair, Matthew snapped. 'Stop asking about my mum's hair. She looks great!' Aw, my son. Bravely leaping to my defence and protecting me from imagined hurt. It worked too... Brodie never mentioned it again, and we had a very happy holiday, complete with birthday tea, which was every bit as special as my 40$^{th}$ had been, now a distant memory in a very long, very traumatic year.

> **Happy birthday Sonja! Hope you have a lovely day and are having a great holiday. Rachel X**

> **Hey, happy birthday old-timer! Have a good one. Gav X**

> **Happy birthday Sonja! I hear from Graham you're celebrating in Loch Tay – sounds like fun. Sister-in-law Big Emma (Switzerland)**

While I was busy enjoying myself - cycling, reading, chatting and having fun, just as the doctor ordered - the Bling Fling organisation was gathering pace.

Four hundred women had now registered, many of them had set up online sponsorship pages and the money was coming in fast. Both Lesley and Lisa were endlessly adding to lists, checking totals, banking money, and dealing with the occasional query... until those two blissful weeks in Loch Tay. I say blissful, because for me it was – I'm not sure that is quite the word Lisa might have used about those Easter holidays shenanigans however....

I must confess that the problems had begun a week before, when the t-shirts arrived..... and we excitedly tore open the boxes and held up the bright pink fabric within.

The logo was there – Bling Fling Tiaras and Trainers Walk instantly recognisable, standing out white and bright on the background of fuschia which had been carefully selected in our weeks of planning.

All was well ... until we tried them on. Picking up a medium, which I had optimistically chosen for myself, I realised that to cram myself into its slimfit style would be comparable to shoving a couple of bowling balls into a corset – and I'm not particularly well endowed.

Between us, our committee covers a range of shapes and sizes, and not one of us was comfortable in the smaller sizes. The horror dawned ... the t-shirts were tiny, and we had no time left to do anything about it.

And so the decision was made, we'd hand them out, matching sizes to order, and hope for the best that people weren't too worried about body image and would be willing to display their wares in the tightest, pinkest T-shirts in town. Some might even choose to go for the distraction technique and use their imagination to rustle up something that would disguise the no secrets-fit - bling was the order of the day, and tight-fitting t-shirts encrusted in diamante would be a perfect antidote to the muffin tops which would no doubt be worrying our girly walkers.

As holder of the Bling Fling phone, Lisa bore the brunt of the Great T-Shirt Disaster, as it came to be known, and while I rested in Loch Tay, she fielded phone call after phone call from women hoping to exchange their shirt for a bigger size, and became an expert of Blue Peter proportions on giving ideas for enhancing and adjusting the too-small shirts, with not a bit of double sided sticky tape in sight...

**Holy shit Sonja!! I just got my Bling Fling t-shirt. I look like a bright pink muscle man! I barely fit into it. Aaargh!**

**Text from my skinniest friend Callum, Gang Show Musical Director and Bling Fling Walker**

## Eliza Cargill, five years old

**My niece Eliza was just starting school when I was diagnosed with breast cancer. She has always appreciated my collection of costume jewellery and sense of style, and probably noticed most the changes in my appearances as I progressed through my cancer treatment. When I asked her what she thought my changing style, she was happy to talk in the straight no-holds-barred way she has down to a tee.**

"The worst thing was when mummy told us that Auntie Sonja had breast cancer. I didn't really know what it was to start with, but mummy said Auntie Sonja was going to go to hospital because there was something wrong with her, and I got really sad.

I also remember mummy telling me and my brothers that Auntie Sonja was going to have chemotherapy which I was scared about because I knew it would make Auntie Sonja's hair fall out. She's always had really long hair, I thought it was really beautiful. I didn't want it to fall out. That made me sad.

She came to the caravan with us when she first got breast cancer and she looked just the same. That weekend, we read the book called Mummy's Got A lump, which was kind of sad but it did explain everything to us. It was sad because I knew all those things were going to happen to Auntie Sonja and that was a shame.

I told my teacher at school and I did cry when I was telling her. But school did make me happy because nobody really knew about it, and I was able to have lots of fun with my friends.

The only difference was when Auntie Sonja got her wig on. But the wig was lovely, and Auntie Sonja looked the same, just as glamorous. My Auntie Sonja always looks glamorous. She wears lovely make-up and jewellery, and I like her clothes and dangly ear rings.

When she stopped wearing her wig, her hair was really short and I didn't really like it. I think it was just a shock when I saw it, because she looked a bit like a boy. But she still wore her lovely clothes and ear rings and always had lip stick on, so she didn't look like a boy really.

Now her hair is growing longer again, and it is curly. It looks really funky and I like it. Now Auntie Sonja wears hairbands and she still looks glamorous. I'm glad she's all better now.

## Chapter 24

**Was thinking about you last night ...
Hope all goes well today. Gav**

The break from treatment over Easter was a welcome one, and gave the chance for my wounds to heal and my body to build up its resources for the third and final step, radiotherapy.

I knew this would be the biggest commitment – time wise, at least. Every day for five weeks, I would make my way up to the hospital for a blast in the giant machines that were so toxic that the people working with them have to stay out of the way at all times when they are doing their damaging stuff.

I'd heard of people being burnt by radiotherapy, skin damaged for life, and I had also been warned that my skin, fair skinned and sun sensitive as it is, may have fared worse under the treatment.

As I have found all the way along, however, what you hear and read about are the worst case scenarios, written and told to you so that you are prepared for the worst – and if the outcome is better than the worst, it is a bonus.

Sandy recently observed that 'the trouble with me is that I always expect the best and so I'm often disappointed'. Whereas in her case she expects the worst and is often pleasantly surprised... in her world, I suppose, that is a good summing up of the glass half full, glass half empty philosophy.

She's right in that I am a glass half full kind of girl. I also don't foresee or imagine problems before they appear, and my soul lives entirely in the moment, making it possible for me to have no real anxieties about radiotherapy. My only concern was for tackling the hospital car parks daily, as parking, as I've mentioned, is never a given right no matter how desperate you are.

The radiotherapy suite is by far the most recently decorated part of the hospital's cancer treatment facilities – the decorator's daughter in me strikes again, living up to the title of Wallpaper Heiress, foisted on me by a journalist colleague many years ago and which still raises a smile at the memory. Pine flooring, coffee tables, plants and soft chairs adorn the clinic's waiting area, giving it – and therefore patients - the feeling of walking into a health spa or beauty parlour. As I got into the routine of radiotherapy over the weeks of whistle-stop visits, and caught up with the daily chat of the radiotherapists while baring my all under the giant machines, I began to believe the illusion I had created for myself that I was indeed going for a daily top-up on a massive sunbed. Not too dissimilar from the reality in fact.

Before the radiotherapists set their powerful assortment of ray guns to work, however, the oncologist had to work out where the dose should be administered, measuring and marking exactly the position while I lay bare breasted – again (fighting breast cancer is not a game for the modest or faint-hearted, you'll be beginning to realise) under a huge scanning machine.

There they marked me up with very thick marker pen, drawing a square like a target onto my breast for the final doses administered straight onto the scar in the final stages of radiotherapy. Called the electron "boost", this is a very superficial beam of radiation aimed straight onto where the tumour was, and is less penetrating than the other radiotherapy, but which may cause my skin to become pinker than the rest. In my case, as they marked up the square, they apologised that they would 'have to take in my nipple too – sorry about that'. Sorry? Well I guess if there was an alternative, they would have done that so really, after filling me full of toxic drugs and cutting into my beloved breast, a few rays on my nipple is the least of my worries. But apology accepted nonetheless...

Once the pen had been drawn came the really anarchic bit – I had to get tattoos (or tatts if you say it in rock chick lingo, as I was tempted to do from time to time for comic effect). Not on my knuckles, as was suggested by a Facebook friend who thought the letters BLING FLING would work well – not as a guide for the radiotherapists, but as an advertising campaign for the walk which by that time had taken over our lives.

The tattoos were actually tiny and very insignificant, but the pin pricks of blue ink were perfectly positioned to be lined up with the machinery, ensuring that I lay in the same position each time the radiation was administered, so the dose would enter my body in exactly the same way, ensuring that maximum impact would be had with little damage to the surrounding area.

Finally, just before I put on my lovely white bra to soak up all the blue ink (which incidentally would never come out, no matter how many washes it went through – didn't bode well for my skin, I thought. I feared I may inherit Lorraine's nickname before the day was out) and headed home for a shower to undo the aforementioned damage, I had to pose for another photograph. This time the photographs of my breast, complete with all the markings, would be used as a reference for the final electron boost which would conclude my course of radiotherapy.

> **Thinking about you getting zapped...**
> **hope all goes well the morn.**
> **Text from Gavin**

The following day, the regime started. Drive to hospital, park in short stay car park (usually a manageable feat, although the one day I abandoned the car, of course, was the one day that the car broke down and I became stuck, fighting back tears of frustration for an hour on the double yellows before by some quirk of fate, it leapt into life. My car has to be a woman – it never lets you down in a crisis). A quick trip into the Clinic, daily chat with the lady who was in for treatment before me, catch-up on the Bling Fling latest with the radiotherapists while I removed my clothes and they admired my latest bra... and then onto the sunbed (as I had nicknamed it, and was now calling it glibly whenever I referred to it) for a quick zapping.

The thing with radiotherapy is that it's not really designed to be comfortable... nor is it particularly warm, which I found somewhat surprising, given that I had thought the sunbed likeness might require me to need protective glasses for the occasion.

What you do is this... you lie down on a bed, bottom in exactly the same place every day, shoulders lying at the same angle, pushed and prodded into place by the obligatory cold hands of the radiotherapist. The position isn't easy either - one hand rests above your head wrist held in place by a stirrup, while your head itself looks away, held in place, unmoving, for around 60 seconds while the fans whir high overhead. Suddenly the machine springs into motion, the treatment bed rises and moves you under the machine in a threatening, claustrophobic inducing fashion – like the Day of the Triffids, the monsters bending in for a closer look.

One radiotherapist sets the treatment machine using numbers and information displayed on a computer screen, projected onto the wall (which as the patient you are absolutely forbidden to look at, holding yourself firmly in pose so that all the good work done placing you does not go awry with one tiny wiggle of nosiness. The other one with the cold hands checks you are not moving and chants numbers to confirm all is set. They check and double check the first position of the Triffid or linear accelerator (its correct title), which delivers the radiation beam from one side of your breast. After the first beam is given the Triffid is moved to the other side of your breast and the same happens again.

Before the first zap they put on the iPod with it's strange and interesting selection of music – everything from Meat Loaf to Daniel O'Donnell represented – flick the lights on, and leave you lying there, cold, terrified to move and holding your breath, knowing that by breathing, you might somehow perhaps dislodge your positioning.....

Then you wait... and still holding that freeze, you wait some more ... and ... to be honest, the whole thing is a huge anticlimax. Given the immense size and complexity of the machinery, I would have expected at least one small teleportation of myself Star Trek style, or a flash of lightning as visible evidence that something was going on.

But the gentle whirring of a fan, followed by a succession of beeps, ending with one long one (like the Morse code, although I'm not really sure what it would have said had I been able to interpret it ... One Wrong Move and the Armpit Gets It or something similar, I should imagine) is all the evidence you get of the radiation entering the cancer boxing ring.

At the end of the long beep, there's a moments' silence when you can start to relax (well, into the fourth week, once I knew the treatment was all over by this point, I started to relax. Up to that point I lay rigid until told by the radiotherapist that I could move) and then the machinery whirred and parted above you, returning to its original overhead position, the bed lowered, so you didn't have to do a pole vault to hit the floor, and you dressed and returned to normal life – no worse of the 15 minutes' hospital visit, until the next day when you returned to go through the whole process again.

It was the radiotherapist who taught me a very important lesson about making people feel good. As I lay in position, prodded to move my buttocks down the bed, my shoulder up, my chin round 'just a tiny bit, too far, there', followed by 'Perfect, that's the perfect position, well done...'

I burst with pride that I could hold the perfect position, I almost wanted them to take a photograph of me holding that perfect position so I could brag about it on Facebook, and I realised the importance of praising people when they are doing well.

The simple task of striking a perfect pose under the radiation machines, which I had done every day for six weeks, made me glow inside – because I had done it 'perfectly'. Gold stars all round.

**Hi Sonja, Thinking of you on the last day of radiotherapy. Lots of Love Lupin, Bling Fling Photographer**

For six weeks I went to the clinic for my daily zapping, diligently massaging Aqueous Cream afterwards to combat the drying effects of the radiation on my skin. For weeks after, I continued the massage process as I had been told, as the radiation continues to work long after the course is complete. Even now I must watch that area of skin in the sun, and spent last summer putting sunblock on the area to stop the new skin becoming damaged by the sun's dangerous UV rays.

Often during radiotherapy I felt a prickling sensation and hotness – something akin to mild sunburn, and my skin took on a pinkish tinge which perfectly matched the Bling Fling t-shirts which by now had been hand delivered and blinged up by every tiara and trainers clad walker in the North-east.

Radiotherapy had indeed been a pussycat of a ride for me, and, ending as it did, three days after the Bling Fling, it became a tiny and familiar routine in my constantly busy day....

How would I cope when the whole merry-go-round of my life stopped? When the hospital routine had ended, the constant bustle of the Bling Fling bubble had burst and I was left free-falling, grabbing for the support network of my family and friends who by that time had done all they could and had to return to their own lives.

The next journey had just begun – and for me, the return to normality was the most difficult road I had travelled yet. But once more I wouldn't be doing it alone ...

**All done friends! Last radiotherapy over. Have a drink on me tonight. Thanks for all your support over the last six months. Couldn't have done it without you.
Text to friends, Sonja**

**Hooray! Great to hear it's all over. You've been so brave and achieved so much... Text from Catriona, Friend**

**Wow! It's amazing all you've been through and it's all done. Hard to believe. You must feel so chuffed. I can't imagine how it feels...**

**Text from Ailsa, neighbour and friend**

# Radiotherapist's Story

Martin Rudge has been a friend of mine since my teenage performing days – he still sings on the amateur stage, and joined us as an entertainer at the Bling Fling. He has also worked as a radiotherapist in Aberdeen for 26 years, and is currently an Imaging Superintendent. When Martin heard I had started chemotherapy, he was there before my second appointment to check out my new wig, and present me with a bagful of magazines suggested for my perusal by his female colleagues. He told me at the time that if I gritted my teeth and bore out the chemotherapy course, by the time I got to radiotherapy it would be a breeze. "We are pussycats compared to these guys," he said. Martin was good as his word when he was there to welcome me to the pamper parlour (as I saw it) at the beginning of my radiotherapy course and told me I looked great with my new very short elfin cut... He told me about the radiotherapists' role in the cancer battle.

"Most ladies have an understanding about Radiotherapy before they arrive in the department. During the planning process we try and explain as much as possible to alleviate any worries or concerns about the treatment. We have information leaflets to refer to in case they do not understand anything, because the first appointment can be quite daunting for some. It's that fear of the unknown. Often ladies request to see the machines before they start. We also try and do our best with appointment times to make the treatment go smoothly for them.

With regards to skin advice, we always prepare breast ladies for the worst case scenario because anything else is actually a bonus. It's far better to warn someone about what could potentially go wrong with their skin, rather than say 'Nothing is going to happen' and suddenly everything erupts, their skin breaks down and they're left saying 'Why didn't you warn me about that?'

It does happen, no matter what type of skin people have, their recovery depends on the skin repair mechanism. You can have a fair-skinned person who might react mildly, and another who will react quite severely. For some, because radiotherapy has an accumulative effect, the worst reaction can develop post treatment, which can be quite a worrying time. We give everyone a helpline number so if there are any problems, they have someone to call for reassurance or support."

The radiotherapy treatment after a mastectomy is slightly different, explains Martin. "The aim of our treatment is to make sure the scar achieves the maximum dose prescribed, so we put on a piece of false tissue on top of the mastectomy scar called bolus, which draws the radiation dose up towards the skin's surface, sometimes causing quite a brisk skin reaction. Unfortunately you can find the worst reaction develops on mastectomy scars rather than those who have had lumpectomies.

"Our job is technically driven, operating the Star Trek/Triffid machines as Sonja calls them, but we are also trained to deal with the many other aspects of patient care and support during treatment. We are very aware as professionals that everyone is an individual and has different needs and we endeavour to help in any way we can.

"Nowadays there is far more support for women going through breast cancer treatment, but it's still a huge emotional journey for women to go through.

As radiotherapists we are sometimes the first to see the scars of surgery and undressing can be a bit upsetting for some, but I would say the majority of women by time they reach us, have been through so much they tend to leave their modesty on the doorstep and pick it up on the way back out again.

If they are worried about it we will do our best to help in any way we can. We've tried all sorts of scenarios to help make it easier. We've had dedicated gowns but the ladies felt they were being pointed out so we stopped that. We've tried screens and not all women want that either. If there's a certain individual who would like to change into a dressing gown, they can do so, but most people are happy by this stage to just get on with it and get through the treatment."

### After Radiotherapy

"Towards the end of Radiotherapy, time is spent in preparing the patient for what happens next. A lot of patients, when they finish radiotherapy, expect to be told "That's it, you're cured, away you go!" but of course there's the whole round of follow-ups and mammograms if required, to come. I think some women have high expectations from the first review appointment after treatment, and

I always tell them 'It's a sort of hello, how are you doing and goodbye review, with all the other surgical and radiographic appointments to follow'. We often see some ladies before their first follow up who have contacted the helpline regarding skin issues.

"Doctors will see women for up to five years or even longer if requested, until they are discharged from the clinic, and most find that so reassuring. A lot of ladies worry the week before their check-up, because you may think it's all over but you're still on that journey. From the day of diagnosis onwards, every little twinge or twitch will bring the thought that the cancer may have come back. It is so important for reassurance and continuing support to be given from all disciplines involved."

### Coping With Radiotherapy

"Cancer crosses all walks of life, and I've seen many women who work during their treatment and who sail through because they've got lots going on, they have partners and families keeping them going. Some are exhausted with trying to keep on top of everything. There are others who might sit at home and mull over everything, everything becomes a problem, and the cancer just highlights the problems. Everyone is different and has a different way of coping.

Some require constant support, others simply do not see the need for it.

"I often view patients with breast cancer as unwell, rather than ill because the majority look so well. Physically most women do look well and I think that makes it harder for some, because people around them will be saying 'You're looking great, but mentally they're maybe finding it very hard."

"The most visible aspect, apart from the hidden scars, for women to cope with is losing their hair as a result of the chemotherapy, so when we compliment them on how they look with their new wig or hair growth – and some women do look great with short hair – they are surprised and delighted. It's given them a new image and it really suits them. For some it's a new beginning. We always check that no one leaves the treatment room with a squint wig!"

## Friendship and fun

"We find at radiotherapy that ladies often meet other people going through the same journey in the waiting room, and that is a good support for some. The machine where Sonja was treated is used mainly for breast work, so most of the ladies going there are being treated for breast cancer. Many women chat while they're waiting and they love to get any niggles sorted out together, by giving each other advice and sharing experiences. That's how some women cope with their illness, talking can be so therapeutic."

## Inner strength

There are some patients who Martin treats who sadly don't have the same sunny outlook as I did by the time they arrive at radiotherapy.

He says: "I still have a lot of empathy and admiration for palliative patients, the ones who know that they're not going to going to be cured and to them life is so precious because time is the issue. You see that on a daily basis in this job. It can be very humbling."

"You can take ten women and some will respond to the treatment and some won't, some will and then relapse ten years down the line. There are many brave women, keeping themselves going to see their child go to school, their daughter get married, their son graduate – it's a focus for them. That will power keeps them going and I think that shows great inner strength, with everything that's going on, they're still able to fight to see their final wish fulfilled.

Martin was also very keen to mention that while he has referred to women undergoing treatment that men too can also develop breast cancer. It can be very difficult for men to come to terms with such a diagnosis because it is so predominately a female one.

## Doing it With Bling On

While I was going through Radiotherapy, I was also hard at work planning the Bling Fling, and one day I persuaded Martin to join us to lend his vocal skills at the Winter Gardens party. As well as thrilling the crowds, he also persuaded many of our Flingers to take to the mike.

He remembers: "The Bling Fling was great and I loved being involved in it. I think it was a positive celebration of Sonja. What impressed me was how she managed to co-ordinate it all while going through treatment as well. The support she had from so many friends and that all those people were willing to do things for her. I think that says a lot about her as a person rather than what she was going through.

"She was able to get so many people involved. I honestly think Sonja would be able to persuade anybody to do anything! It was a real pleasure and a privilege to be part of it."

# Chapter 25

The day before the Bling Fling the heavens opened... rain poured from the grey leaden skies, ran along the pavements, collected around the blocked drains and threatened to flood the streets around the Duthie Park – the one place we had hoped the sun would shine on our intrepid walkers.

Even the worst May weather Aberdeen had seen in years did nothing to deter Pam and her husband Andrew from carrying out their Bling Fling duties, intrepidly setting out on bikes along the Railway Line to hammer direction signs into the already subsiding ground. With their children in tow, the four became our answer to Noah's doves, flying out in the torrents to mark the way for our walkers, and checking out Lisa's much-requested toilets which were by now installed at the halfway point, before heading back to base with their olive branch information in situ.

The rest of us spent the morning dropping off wine at the park – 280 bottles of pink fizz to be precise, and collecting tables and chairs which had been delivered to nestle amongst the greenery of the lush Winter Gardens the following evening, while stage manager Judith and her stage crew were busily employed setting up the stage and sound system in readiness for the party.

In other words, everyone was working tirelessly to bring the day to fruition.... only the weather, it seemed, was failing to hold up its end of the bargain.

Not that we were worried about a bit of rain, however ... in our book, no self-respecting pink, bling-clad Aberdonian would ever let the grey wet stuff get in the way of party. It was not until a phone call came through from the council that the concerns really began to set in. "What are your contingency plans if this rain continues?" said the sensible suit-wearing voice on the end of the line. "Are you going to cancel – because we suggest that you do. There may be health and safety issues if you go ahead..."

What?... cancel? After all this effort, all this fundraising – we already had £23k pledged on our Just Giving site, and everything was full speed ahead for the following day. How could we cancel – and what's more, why should we? I mean, inclement weather is hardly an oddity in our colourful North-east world in which every season can be represented in one day...

We spoke about it, sounded out Pam and Andrew who had already seen the line – and were our Health and Safety supremos remember (sorry Pam, but much as she hates being known as such, it is honestly a skill I greatly admire in her, and her knowledge of such things intrigues me as though it were something of a magical power) – and they pointed out that the line had a hard surface and was therefore unlikely to fall away in a rain-induced land slide. The Bling Fling would go ahead regardless – we just had to hope that our specially designed T-shirts decorated with as much bling as the Aberdeen branch of John Lewis could possibly throw at them - would be seen under the mountain of raincoats and brollies which would inevitably ensue if the weather continued.

Fiona had arrived from London the Saturday before the Bling Fling, and we spent that evening together, eating curry and sheltering from the rain in a restaurant we had dived into on the way into town, unprepared to get any wetter on our search for good food. We talked, and laughed, and distracted ourselves from the torrents pouring down outside, refusing to think of the rivulets that were probably forming on the old railway line as we ate.

By the time I went to bed that night, I was cold and wet, my excitement for the following day replaced with trepidation about what we do with the 400 bling-covered drowned rats who would crawl back to the Winter Gardens at the end of the walk, needing cocoa and a hot bath more than the gallons of pink fizz we had amassed over the weeks of preparation.

My single abiding thought as I struggled to sleep that night was 'Why oh why didn't we organise waterproof ponchos – just in case?'

The weather forecast was for more of the same, the rain would continue - and so it was with a heavy heart that I lay awake into the wee small hours, trying to sleep, hoping against hope for a miracle in which a happy little sun would somehow settle over Ferryhill for just long enough for the Bling Fling to take place...

**Yippee! It's not raining! Here's to a fabulous day ladies ... thanks in advance for the last few months and for being there. You are truly great friends, Sonja X**

**Hi, thanks Sonja. You are a great motivator. Lovely day – so excited! See you all soon, Lisa X**

**It's going to be a great day. You too are a great friend. Janine X**

If I ever doubted someone up there was looking down on us, I took it all back on Sunday 17th May 2009. The battering torrents of overnight seemed to vanish as the sun came up, drying everything in an instant and bathing Aberdeen in the glitter that adorns granite on a summer's day. Even the city seemed blinged up for the occasion.

I remember sitting in Lisa's garden that morning as text after text came in, claiming that 'the sun shines on the righteous', 'someone was looking after us', and 'a small miracle has occurred', and I have to say they were right. That sudden weather change hardly ever happens in Aberdeen, and for the sun to shine as brightly and for as long after days of torrential rain, we were indeed indebted to a far greater force than our own positive thoughts.

As Lisa and I drank tea, laughed excitedly and spoke about it feeling like a wedding day – only with six brides, all as excited as the next and able to share that excitement between us.

**It will be a busy day but it will be great. Enjoy! See you later, Ailsa X**

Ailsa was absolutely right with this text message on the morning of the Bling Fling – it was to be the busiest day in memory – but worth every minute of the blood, sweat and tears we had poured into the day.

The morning saw us gathered at the park, depositing food and setting up tables for the evening event. At lunchtime, our friends from the Gang Show arrived to pitch the tent which would provide shelter for the registration team, and the outdoor stage and sound system was set in place for the mass blinged up workout which was to follow.

It's hard to describe how I felt that afternoon, as hundreds of women – some family and old friends, others strangers attracted by the chance to wear a tiara and raise money for the Bling Fling charities, or just keen to have a fun afternoon at Aberdeen's newest girly event – gathered on the grass in the sunshine, ready to take the Old Deeside Line by storm.

We started into the day with £23k in our account – the result of online donations, sponsorship by local companies, and various fundraisers in the run up to the event. One of our walkers had come up with the idea of hosting a Cocktails and Cupcakes night at her home – at which we were special guests - and invited 60 friends to bring and buy home-bakes and a raffle prize, raising a whopping £1,000 for the Bling Fling charities and setting herself a hard act to follow when she restaged the event for the Bling Fling Christmas Thing later in the year.

Volunteers joined us from the charities themselves, local shops, friends and family members – including my dear old dad who led up the counting team, and banked all the money brought along on the day. A job to which he was perfectly suited, loved every minute of and gave him the chance to dress in a pink jumper I had never seen before but he claims has been in his wardrobe for years.

Four hundred walkers turned up and swamped the park in bling, the money and pledges came rolling in, and we chattered excitedly, swapping girly gossip, greeting people we had known for years, introducing ourselves to those we had just met, and feeling genuinely inspired by the efforts some had made to be there, and had spent in kitting themselves out in the cause of our tiaras and trainers theme.

Taking the stage to give my carefully rehearsed opening speech (I say carefully rehearsed as I had read it to all who would listen in the run-up to the event, so that when speaking from the heart and therefore letting some very raw emotion surface, I would not be tempted to cry while opening such a fun-packed event), I looked out on the sea of pink before me and along at the row of my special friends who shared with me the platform and the glory of the day. As I took in the scene, I remember thinking, once again, how lucky I was - to be almost finished my cancer treatment, to have shared the journey with such fabulous friends, and now to have shared the experience of organising an event as great and as life-changing as the Bling Fling would ultimately be.

Graham was recording the Bling Fling on video, while another couple of friends were our official photographers, and I was given the fun job of chauffeuring the snappers along the line to grab photos at the important points en route – I think this was possibly as an attempt to keep me out of the way while the more talented list-makers and organisers on our team got busy setting up the food and party for the returning walkers, but whatever the reason, it gave me the chance to do what I do best and chat to our band of walkers, cheering them on as they paced the 10km path back to the awaiting party.

When photographer Lupin joined me on an old bridge traversing the line, we looked down together on the walkers, snaking into the distance, a veritable pink river flowing beneath us, singing and dancing in the sunshine. She turned to me and said 'You must feel really proud... this is your army Sonja – your own pink army...' She must have read my thoughts... proud was exactly the word I would have used to describe how I felt at that moment. Proud of everything we had achieved and were achieving in the miraculous sun of that early summer evening.

Returning to the park after completing the amble (I always gave walkers the instructions to walk at chatting speed – an idea a friend suggested might catch on if I invented a walking machine encompassing exactly that girly speed suggested), my fellow organisers in Bling had readied the botanical gardens to house the after walk party. Entertainers and therapists were secreted away among the plants in every available space, topless cowboys lined up to pour the 298 bottles of pink fizz for the weary walkers and the canapés and copious amounts of chocolate were plated up and ready to pleasure (still not quite enough, but I doubt you'd ever get it spot on when estimating the amount of chocolate a crowd of girls will consume if tired and merrily on their way to snoozeville after exercise and a fun night out with friends).

Wandering into the Winter Gardens, full of stovies and high on life, the Bling Fling ladies were met by a glass of fizz, canapés and the sounds of a string quartet drifting through the orangerie style glasshouses of the Silver City's tropical paradise.

Walking through the Victorian glass corridors, walkers came upon dancers, Rat Pack singers, fashions shows, barbershop choruses, fashion shows and various therapists offering hand, head and feet massages, nail painting, hair advice, and the very important Breast Awareness tips.

At the end of the evening, everyone gathered to sing New York New York round the piano, 500 voices lending their support to our cause and celebrating life and friendship at the end of a tumultuous year.

The evening of the Bling Fling, we announced that so far we had raised £51,000 to be shared between our three charities. Later that figure rose to £73,000 as sponsor money came in long after the evening itself. The pride of handing these life-changing totals to our three charities over the next six weeks was immense, and brought home to us the achievement and dedication of the Bling Fling walkers whose support had made the event a success and our dreams a reality in this first fantastic year.

As the party ended, our committee watched everyone leave, a flurry of bling heading out into the darkness, then found a picnic table at which to sit outside enjoying the calm and still of the warm evening, high on success, high on life and high on friendship, sharing a few bottles of pink fizz as we digested the day's events. We wanted it to go on forever, and if it couldn't do that, to bottle the feeling the Bling Fling had stirred up and keep it for a dull moment in the future to be taken out and treasured all over again...

When the wind chill finally got to us all, we headed for the nearest hotel, willing the night to last as long as possible, and met up with a barful of girls wearing the instantly recognisable slightly too tight pink T-shirts which had become the bane of our lives for the few weeks leading up to the walk.

As we arrived, hailed as heroes and offered drinks from several grateful well wishers, the chat turned to what would we do next... someone suggested a Christmas Ball, setting in motion the wheels of our imagination once more...

Six months later, the Bling Fling Christmas Thing was launched, raising another £8,000 for our chosen charities, another fun-packed night for 400 women and a chance for me to meet many more friends of friends and strangers up to that point, who were at different stages of their cancer journey, each taking comfort from that fun night spent with friends which would go a little way to encouraging them to Do It With Bling On, battling cancer in whatever way they could and harnessing the support they could from those around them .

A few memories stand out in the wonderful pink haze of that first ever Bling Fling – and one of them is meeting Audrey. Audrey was diagnosed with breast cancer around the same time as I was. She was aged 39, mum of a five-year-old little boy, wife of her teenage sweetheart and colleague of my friend Lorraine.
Through Lorraine, I had heard of her failed chemotherapy, how her cancer had continued to grow and spread, becoming secondary tumours by the time of the Bling Fling.
I also knew that she'd embraced the whole Tiaras and Trainers concept from the minute it was first suggested, encouraged her friends to join her on the 5km walk (which is all she would manage, her health and strength beginning to take its toll on her usually high energy levels) and found herself on the day smiling, laughing, surrounded by her friends dressed in pink wings and halos, playing their self-assigned role of Audrey's Angels to perfection.
I'd heard all about Audrey's bright personality and positive energy, so to meet her and laugh while she embraced me and told me off for making her cry when I spoke at the opening ceremony provided my most touching moment of that day and one that will surely stick with me forever.

When a couple of months later I stood at her funeral with her friends in their pink Bling Fling T-shirts and listened as they told me that wonderful May day had provided their happiest, brightest memory in those last few months of their young friend's life, was humbling indeed. To see her old dad, sitting in shock, confusedly wondering why he had lost his youngest child so early, knocking the expectations of his life sideways and in so doing, losing the sense of preordained order that being a father should bring. You're not supposed to outlive your children... your grandchildren need their mother, not their grandparent around to watch them grow... there is no sense in a 39-year-old dying and her 80-year-old dad trying to make sense of it at her funeral.

When Audrey died, I had an idea which I ran by the girls on the Bling Fling committee. They agreed with me that a fitting tribute to her wonderful zest for life and commitment to our cause would be to have the Bling Fling research project carried out in her memory. The Prof agreed and we're all hoping that the work currently being funded will take scientists a little closer to working out why some patients respond to chemotherapy and others don't, thus saving precious weeks that could and should save lives.

I feel privileged to have known Audrey for that short but meaningful time and to be able to do something to make sense of her premature death, to find a positive in the sadness, to channel some of her energy and love of life into something that will surely, sometime in the future, save families from going through the anguish of losing a mother, sister, partner and friend to breast cancer.

In a way, as I saw it, Audrey's death gave me even more reason to live my life to the full - to make the most of the fact that I had, by sheer luck, responded to treatment and made it through. I'll never forget it could so easily have been the other way. As I said at the beginning of this story, everything about cancer is random. I was one of the lucky ones who made it - at times I felt guilty about that, it even preyed on my mind a little on the down days, but most of the time I felt grateful, living my life to the full for those who had never been given the chance to...

## Ian Dow, Aberdeen Gang Show Convener, writes after the Bling Fling:

Very well done, an amazing day that I am sure surpassed anything you first thought about. Everyone I asked if they had a good time, were gushing with praise, for the idea and the organisation. The ending was just perfect.

I know Gang Show were there in big numbers, but we all felt it a privilege to be there helping. That is a mark of the love we hold for you Sonja and your friends.

A big, big thank you for asking us to be involved.

## Ian Booth, Aberdeen Gang Show cast, writes

"What a day! It was fantastic - a huge congratulations to you and your team, who organised an amazing day in perfect settings. How you managed to get the weather right is just amazing!

From the time that the marquee was getting set up in the afternoon to the time I saw you walking out as the last person in the Winter Gardens it was all go but so well managed that the time really flew in. All of the ladies I spoke to were hugely complimentary and asking for more of the same next year.

It must have been hugely satisfying for you as well, considering all that you have gone through in the past year.

Once again, Sonja congratulations for what was a wonderful day. The money raised almost seems incidental - but of course that was the real purpose of the day. To have had such a successful day AND raising over £70,000 is simply amazing!!!

# Chapter 26

Throughout the final chapters of this book I've hinted at the fact that it was not all going to be plain sailing... somewhere along the way, I had to have a crash landing it seemed.

Everyone reaches an emotional crisis at a different time in their cancer journey - mine happened after the Bling Fling, at which point I crashed out in style....

It makes sense to me now that it happened when it did. I've always been the kind of person who copes with a crisis while it's happening and then thinks about it when it's nearly over. I remember having a major panic attack just before my University Final exam, when mum sat up with me through the night giving me focuses for my study, and pulling me through my nerves-induced mental block at the last moment ... I always freak out just before a show is set to hit the stage and let fly in diva-like fashion at some poor unsuspecting member of the production team or stage crew...

So it was not wholly unexpected when, as the Bling Fling and radiotherapy came to an end and everyone drifted off back to their own lives, an out-of-control melancholy swept over me like a wave, engulfing me and my world for the next few months. If I'm honest, at that stage I could have run away, crawled into a cave, made a new life for myself far, far away from all those who had seen me through the last few months – moving on seemed far easier than trying to find a way back to where I had come from at that particular time.

I had survived breast cancer, but what was left? Six months before I was a 40-year-old bright strong woman who had unquestioningly enjoyed good health and a happy future among family and friends. Now, six months of pounding by chemotherapy, radiotherapy, surgeons and an emotional journey of gargantuan proportions, I was exhausted and in mourning for the care-free life I appeared to have lost somewhere along the way.

Graham and my family were ready to celebrate – crack open the champagne, pronounce the end of the battle, and head back to the comfortable place we had left the very minute I learned I had breast cancer.

The children were also hopeful of a return to normality, a calm after the storm, and suddenly I felt the obligation to be the person they knew and loved, to find the road back to the me I had left behind, to pick up the pieces of myself I had lost along the way and return to the starting post, a well woman who could be the person I was before, revitalised and with the new lease of life that facing my own mortality would bring.

Of course, I – and they – were expecting too much. It wasn't all going to happen just like that. When I got to the stage that I was angry, lashing out at those around me, accusing them of not being there for me, not supporting me, not understanding what I was going through, I realised that I had travelled this journey as far as I could go in my own way. If I carried on kicking, I would lose the people closest and dearest to me, and the whole battle would be deemed worthless anyway.

It seemed I had lost the map, I was floundering alone in a mist of my own making and I had to get myself back onto the pathway of my life before I could set off again and rejoin my family and friends on the way.

Whether or not I could ever go back to where I had set out from on that fateful August day was unclear and unlikely, but to restart my journey, I had to stop battling against those around me and calmly find an inroad to bring me closer to them again and thereby merge the roads we had all been following before my initial diagnosis.

With this conclusion, I did as I have done all the way through my cancer year and headed for CLAN, to make use of another of its facilities – counselling. There I met Graeme, a counsellor, who became my confidante and friend, who helped me to begin and continue the final journey – back to emotional wellbeing – which for me seemed the longest and hardest road of all.

I still remember sitting in the counsellor's room on that first day as Graeme came out with the line I would cling onto – "Some people describe this feeling as having been led by the hand through cancer treatment, and then falling off a cliff when it's all over."
At the time I told him that I didn't feel I had been led by the hand through treatment – I had, in fact, done a lot of the hand-holding and most often led the way for those around me. But yes, I agreed that the feeling I was currently experiencing felt like the result of dropping from a great height. A long and exhilarating freefall, during which I realised I had forgotten to pack a parachute to soften the blow.

Over the next few months, we met often to chat through my latest personal crisis as Graeme listened and without standing judgement on what I had to say, helped me unravel the thoughts and feelings that had collected or become tangled over the previous months. I knew very well I had protected everyone around me by shouldering much of my journey myself. Now I had to unburden myself of all that I had taken on so that I could move forward with confidence into my future, whatever that would hold.

I also realised that where my friendships with friends and some family had flourished and strengthened as a result of my cancer battle, there were some relationships that were truly floundering. Graeme revealed, interestingly, that going through something like cancer tests every relationship – strong ones become stronger, but by the same token, if there are cracks, they will be found and can be torn asunder with the onset of a cancer battle.

Admitting to having a problem is hard for me. Admitting to it being my fault is even harder. But truth be told I had gone through treatment in my own, some may say, selfish way, I was supported by those whom I turned to and I withdrew from those who needed my support as I would have struggled to offer it, already pulling on my full resources to get myself and the children through.

Hours of chat with the counsellor have shown me that I did what I had to do to cope with my cancer journey, and those around me did the same. You think because you are married to someone, or they have grown up with you or even given birth to you, you will somehow know exactly what is needed to support one another through breast cancer. Sometimes it does come naturally, but most of the time it is a struggle. Not one of us is the same person, we all deal with a crisis differently and a journey like this one can challenge even your closest relationships to the core, revealing strengths and weaknesses both together and individually, and making you realise that years of history symbolises nothing when it comes to the crunch.

You cannot prepare yourself for battling cancer. When it comes down to it, you will fight it in your own way - united you will stand or divided you will fall, and only in the aftermath will you be able to pick up the pieces and try to get it all working again...

My friend Janine said to me recently: "I'd never thought until you came through this what a massive hurdle it is to recover from cancer. Now you probably have 40 years ahead of you like the rest of us, but you also have the experience of having seen your mortality. I don't know how I would cope with that."

The easy way would be to start again, recreate your life in exactly the way you'd want it, making the changes and adjustments to bring you happiness and fulfilment as you deserve. In a way, I suppose I've done that by finding more space in my life – more 'me time' as it were – indulging my interests, delegating my workload, being more choosy as to what I do in my spare time and not feeling as if I need to be everything for everyone. Planning the Bling Fling and writing this book are other steps towards the new more fulfilled Sonja Rasmussen.

But there are basic features of your life you can't change – including your family and children, close relationships which have been through the mill and need lots of time and patient handling to bring them back into line.

A breast cancer diagnosis is like an explosion in the very centre of your world, forcing everything you ever believed you held tightly and most dear rocketing out of reach for a time.

When eventually you land, you can start to pick up the pieces. And finally, and with very careful handling, you will manage to fit them back together – perhaps not in the same pattern, often with a different emphasis on what's important, but someday they will slide into place and become your life again.

# Counsellor at Clan

**Graeme has been a counsellor at CLAN for almost four years. I asked him about the role counselling plays in the cancer battle.**

"It is difficult to make generalisations about how people deal with cancer since each experience is highly subjective. Also, it goes without saying that there is a broad spectrum of diagnoses with some fortunate people having excellent outcome and others being not so lucky. That being said, there are, in my experience, some common themes.

Firstly I never cease to be surprised by the courage and strength that people generally find when faced with cancer. Secondly, the onset of cancer can, in many circumstances, instigate a process of change to occur within a person. Without going into detail, this may involve a change in their outlook on life, their priorities and, in some cases, their sense of self.

My training as a counsellor was in the Person-Centred approach. Basically, this approach deems the client and not the counsellor to be the expert in the client's life. The counsellor does not lead the client nor advise him or her. The idea is to engage with, and where appropriate, support the client in their time of need. The intention is to form a relationship of two equal people meeting for a common purpose in which trust is developed and a deep level of sharing takes place. Often this can lead to meetings at what is sometimes called 'rational depth', where two people are sharing at a deep and meaningful level of understanding and communication, which does not commonly happen in other professional relationships.

Whilst I regularly share a client's feelings and experiences at a deep level, there is always a quality of detachment in my involvement in that sharing process. I try to understand, or more accurately empathise with what the client is feeling but I cannot allow myself to be fully drawn into that experience so that I become overwhelmed by it. If it were otherwise, I could not do my job.

Similarly, because I remain a stranger to the client outside the counselling relationship, the client and I do not run the risk of offending each other. Instead, the relationship encourages a complete openness and sharing, free of fears of upsetting each other. The same cannot be said for other relationships such as those with loved ones or friends, where there often has to be a deep restraint around what the client can share with such persons. This kind of professional detachment, along with empathy, openness or 'realness' and compassionate warmth on the counsellor's part, are often considered to be the main strength of counselling.

As counsellors we deal with very serious issues on a day-to-day basis. That is not to say, however, that humour is not often evident within our centre itself or even at times within the counselling relationship. At CLAN there is an ethos of positivity and optimism mixed in with caring warmth – humour and laughter are often heard within the building. At times humour and laughter can, of course, be very therapeutic in themselves.

At the risk of sounding clichéd, I would like to add that is an immense privilege to work with clients who repose an abiding trust in me and who never fail to hold my interest with their courage, humanity, unique specialness and frankness. This is the reward that I receive from doing this type of work and it will be obvious to the reader that such experiences are not commonplace in the everyday work environment.

Sonja's sense of humour, vigour and optimistic, cheerful personality shine through in this book and it has been rewarding to me to have met her and shared a small part of her story. My thanks go out to her for all the support she has given to CLAN.

We at CLAN are deeply indebted to the generosity of Sonja and the many others like her who give unselfishly of their time and energy in supporting a very important cause."

# Afterword

When I was thinking about how to end this book, I had a problem... Where to finish? With my last radiotherapy? The Bling Fling? The Bling Fling Christmas Thing?

But then I got to the end of each of these experiences and a whole new chapter sprang up, a problem to be overcome, a challenge to be beaten and I realised that the truth is that my cancer story has not ended. My treatment is finished, some day my check-ups and mammograms will also end. But my story, like my life, goes on.

If someone dies of cancer, there is an ending of sorts – people can look back at their life, at their battle and have their own memories. Of course, those they leave behind continue their story, but there is a conclusion.

When someone survives cancer, as I have done, there is no ending. There's just a new beginning... every day at the moment is my new beginning, filled with the challenges and adventure that every new day brings.

I still run towards self-imposed finishing lines, face up to the sun, laughing all the way, and I think I always will do...

My life is a work in progress, my cancer journey was a wrinkle in time, filled with memories both happy and harrowing, challenging and inspirational.

Just as I met people who amazed me with their courage and positivity throughout the last year, so I still meet, and will continue to meet those people who make this world a special place and my life a breath-taking adventure.

And so I leave you with your own story, on the brink of the rest of your life, as I am with mine. Poised, happy, ready for whatever comes next, living in the moment, enjoying and cherishing those around me – and always, especially now, taking the time to fly the kite of my life high and joyously along the way.

<u>Steps to Doing It With Bling On</u>

**You found a lump?**
- Get it checked out! Call your GP FAST...
- Don't panic ... but do everything you can to speed up the process of finding out what's going on. Confide in a close friend...

**Hearing the results and diagnosis**
- Bring a sensible, level-headed friend and a notebook. Hand your friend the notebook and tell them to write down everything the doctor or oncologist tells you. They must ask questions too – because somewhere along the way you'll stop listening and find yourself on the desert island of your dreams
- At the appointment, try to listen to as much as you can, but don't worry if you zone out – that's what you've brought your sensible level-headed friend along for...
- After the appointment is over, and you've had a few hours to recover from the shock of the news, go through your friend's notes with them on hand to discuss and chat things over with you. You'll be amazed at how much you missed and everything will be far clearer and less worrying when you're at home in your own surroundings

**Getting through the initial shock**
- Spend time reading all the booklets and leaflets you are given by the hospital. You will have a few sleepless

nights, so use them wisely by reading and preparing yourself for what lies ahead.
- It is okay to cry and feel sorry for yourself and your family ... but the why me? approach won't make your cancer journey a fulfilling and positive one. Try to go with the view 'Why not me? – I can do this and at the end of it I will be one of the lucky ones who will appreciate who and what is good in my life'
- Spend some time thinking of what makes your life good then go ahead and enjoy it. Immerse yourself in your friendships, spend time with those closest to you, renew old acquaintances who get in touch because they've heard what you're going through, make plans for nights out and weekends away and have fun - this is your chance to indulge yourself. Do it in style!

**Appointments**
- Always bring someone with you – even if they can't come in to appointments, it's nice to have someone there to hold your bling, catch up on the celebrity mags – and tell you about their findings over coffee or lunch afterwards
- It's always more fun if you make an appointment into a social occasion
- Leave yourself enough time to park and get to your appointment – or you could do as I did and always be running late. No time to think about it works too...
- Wear easily accessible clothes – blouses with buttons up the front. This is especially useful when you're going to multiple appointments and having to bare your all in each... It is also necessary if you are wearing a wig at later appointments, so you don't have to do redo your hairstyle each time.

**Telling children**
- Drip feed your children information in the run-up to your final diagnosis. I told mine that I had a lump and the doctor was looking at it with x-rays to see how he would make it go away
- Tell them when you're going to the hospital for final appointments – children are very sensitive and know

when things are going on. It is better not to keep them in the dark entirely
- In the early days, only share the facts with friends you know you can rely on not to speak about it when the children are around. Make sure they will keep it a secret – you don't want your children to hear anything second hand and believe me, they hear everything… especially what they're not supposed to…
- When you first tell them about the cancer, spare them the worst case scenario. I told mine that the doctors had looked at the lump in my breast. They said it was dangerous to leave it as it would grow, and they would need to use strong medicine to make it go away. That medicine was so strong it would make my hair fall out but they could help me choose a nice wig. Always put a positive spin on the news…
- Children will all respond to your diagnosis differently. You know your children best, but with mine, I strived to be normal and bright around them, reassuring them that yes, I was a little scared and I would rather this wasn't happening, but I knew the doctors were very clever at their job and they would do everything they could to make it all better
- If you have young children, make sure you get the book Mummy Has a Lump, from the hospital. Read it a few times out loud before you read it to the children – it is important to stay in control when you are discussing your treatment with them. If they know you are worried, they will realise there is something to worry about - so best get your emotions in check so you don't blub when reading
- Sometimes it is easier to ask someone else to read to them first and answer their questions
- For teenagers, the website TIC – Teen Information on Cancer – is a good one to look up. It explains things really well, it's pitched at the perfect level and there are forums to speak to others, as well as stories and information about all kinds of cancer
- If children ask a question, if it is important enough for them to ask that question, they need an answer to it. Don't fob them off with 'You don't need to worry about

that, we'll take care of that'. There's nothing worse than thinking 'Everyone's in on the secret except me'
- Tell the school and in particular, the children's teachers. They can even bring their book in to share with them. This got my children talking with someone outwith the family unit, and gave them a personal ally in whom they could confide
- The children's group at Clan House is a lifeline for any problems you can't deal with. It also organises days out and special treats to give the children a focus away from family for a while. Some questions and discussion may come out of these experiences which the staff there are very able to deal with.
- Finally, don't given your children any reason to worry... this is a year of their childhood. Give them a year to remember for the good times - the times they spend with you

**For chemotherapy sessions**
- Line up a different friend to come to each session with you – or you could do like a friend of mine did and appoint one special chemo buddy
- Make sure that your chemo buddy knows what's expected of them – providing magazines, crossword puzzles, snacks, lots of celebrity gossip, newsy chat and laughs – and hint that a wee present wouldn't go amiss either!
- Dress up as if you're going for a girlie lunch – look and feel terrific... that always helps!
- If your appointment is later in the day, do something to take your mind off it – window shopping followed by lunch always did the trick for me before chemo
- Be prepared to wait for treatment – and don't be afraid to start the gossip and snacks before the treatment gets underway if they leave you waiting for an hour or more – going away for coffee and coming back when they're ready for you can help to while away the hours
- The best and most useful snacks I found were ginger beer and fresh pineapple, with ginger chocolate and ginger fudge (in small quantities) also proving popular. But be warned – anything you eat in the chemotherapy ward

will never pass your lips again... I know, I've baulked at the sight of pineapple in many a fruit salad since

**After chemotherapy sessions**
- Keep drinking pineapple juice and have a stock of crystallised ginger or ginger biscuits on hand for nausea
- Wear travel bands for a week – they help ward off feelings of sickness too
- Take all the drugs you are given – as my sister told me 'There are no prizes for being a superhero. The important thing is you get through it in one piece'
- Make sure you get a good night's sleep after chemo by taking the anti-sickness drugs prescribed. Don't wait until it's too late – take them as an avoidance strategy
- Don't lie in bed waiting to feel awful – keep getting up every morning and making plans for the day. If you can't face doing them, people will understand, but do everything you can to stay focused and positive
- Although it's not medically proven to help, I stocked up on vitamins during chemotherapy, taking vitamin pills and plenty of fresh fruit and vegetables. I also used an anti bacterial hand gel and nasal spray to guard against infection. Who knows if it worked – but I stayed healthy through a winter of snuffly children and cold-ridden adults so I can only assume it helped a little
- Keep a supply of energy drinks on hand for when you really need a boost – and try to sleep when you need it. Having 40 winks during the day is a guilt-free indulgence you can enjoy during your cancer treatment...

**Coping with the weeks between chemotherapy sessions**
- Whatever you do, don't sit around and feel sorry for yourself...
- Get plenty of fresh air – walks or cycle rides with friends or family are good
- Try to avoid crowded places where you are likely to pick up germs. Flasks at the end of a walk are preferable to crowded coffee shops in the first week after chemotherapy, but coffee shops first thing in the morning (before the

crowds have gathered) are always a treat, chemotherapy or not
- Indulge in daytime cinema trips with a friend, where you will likely be the only ones in the place sharing tissues over a schmaltzy movie, or ogling over a good-looking actor
- If you feel up to it, take a little exercise – yoga or dance class will lift your spirits and help work off the results of the cheese scones you may be indulging in each morning!
- Start reading – my book group was a great source of distraction and gossip when I wasn't out and about as much as usual...
- Invest in a jigsaw puzzle ... always good to focus the mind and while away a quiet moment
- Catch up with friends and take everyone up on their offers. You'll get to know your routine – when you feel well enough to socialise – and book in coffee dates, lunch dates, evenings out, all of which will help make your cancer journey a more enjoyable one.

**Looking good**
- Making sure I always looked my best raised my confidence and mood through cancer treatment. Having people say how great you look is always a boost no matter what you're going through
- Take care over your make-up. You won't have to spend any time on your hair if you're wearing a wig, so use the time instead to make sure your skin, eyes and cheeks are glowing and healthy. Always wear lipstick and pay special attention to your eyes, drawing on eyebrows and sticking on false eyelashes if you lose your own ones
- Choose a wig carefully. Bring a friend whose judgement you trust to help make the decision ... if you can afford to, change your wig halfway through treatment – it feels like you've got a completely new look which is a boost in itself
- Treat yourself to some new underwear – mine was always much admired by the radiographers when I went for radiotherapy. It's lovely to feel you're looking great by the people who are zapping you!

- Glamorous pyjamas are a must for hospital – you may not feel great, but at least you'll look hot to trot while lounging around watching daytime television and eating hospital food
- Buy some nice hats and fab jewellery – charity shops are full of them, and your hair will change so many times over the months, it gives you the opportunity to reinvent your image many times. Bliss!
- Look to CLAN (Cancer Link Aberdeen and North) for support. The support groups are not for everyone – but they offer some lovely therapies including reflexology, aqua detox, relaxation and healing and aromatherapy which are always a treat… time out for yourself is also an important part of CLAN's service
- Keep in touch with people through texting or computer friendship sites like Facebook. You don't have to go over the news time and again with everyone you meet, they can dip in and out of your life and learn what you are up to, and you can respond to them in your own time. The messages you receive will also help support you and make you feel cared about through your treatment

**Friends can be helpful too!**
- If a friend of yours is diagnosed with breast cancer, don't panic or worry what to say
- Of course everyone is different, and you know your friends best, but for me, my friends kept normality going in the midst of everything and that was a very important role
- Suggest walks, coffee, cinema trips, manicures, charity shop trawls – all the things that you like to do as friends CAN and SHOULD still be done
- Always be free enough to have a cup of tea or coffee – or even crack open a bottle of wine. If your friend wants to speak, it should be right then. Don't let the moment pass
- If your friend looks tired or fed up, offer to take their children for a while to let them sleep, put their feet up or go have some me time
- Be willing to go to appointments, to choose a wig, to eat hospital food, to run children's parties…. and do it all

with a smile. Remember your friend is going through a whole lot worse and is depending on you to maintain a sense of well-being and normal life
- Laugh lots – remember funny stories, bits of chat, magical moments and share them. That's what friends are for...
- Make every appointment special by spoiling your friend rotten – she is worth it you know
- Offer to do household chores. A friend offered to clean my toilets, a job I always hate and not just while undergoing chemotherapy, another took ironing away and brought it back looking pressed and beautiful. Yet another took meals round to put in the freezer for an 'off day'. These gifts are precious, practical and mean so much more than a houseful of flowers
- Be there, be strong and be thoughtful. These months will bring many memories and shared experiences that will bond you together forever. Be the positive part of your friend's cancer journey....

**And finally, find things to laugh about ...**
- Laughter is the best medicine after all
- People always find you more attractive and approachable if you smile, and you will find yourself surrounded by friends and support from beginning to end of your cancer treatment
- A cancer diagnosis does not have to be the worst time in your life – you could instead see it as a positive, life-changing and fulfilling experience which will bring your friends and family closer than they've ever been ... and give you time to enjoy those relationships to the full
- Everyone who suffers from and fights cancer, whatever their outcome, is a very special person... I've met many fantastic strong women over the past year whose lives have been changed dramatically by breast cancer treatment... all say life will never be the same again... this is the beginning of a new you. Inspiring, inspirational, awesome. Those of us who have fought breast cancer, can conquer the world...

# Contacts List

## Wigs

Finishing Touches: Phone 01224-211117
info@finishingtouches-wigs.co.uk
29a Ashley Gardens
Aberdeen AB10 6SH
**For readers outwith Aberdeen, information about local wig stockists will be available from your Breast Care Nurse or local treatment centre.**

## Make-Up Advice

Look Good Feel Better Workshop
(Once a month and twice a month alternately)
Aberdeen Royal Infirmary
Foresterhill
Aberdeen
AB25 2BN
Tel: 0845-4566000 ext 59377
**These workshops are available at hospitals throughout the country. Check with your breast care nurse for details information**

## Mummy's Lump

Published by Breast Cancer Care, this book for young children is written by Gillian Forrest and illustrated by Sarah Garson.
It follows the story of brother and sister Jack and Elly, and how they cope with their mummy's diagnosis and treatment of breast cancer. The book covers topics including what Breast Cancer is, what happens at the hospital, the side effects of radiotherapy and chemotherapy, and what will happen after treatment has finished.
It is written and designed in a child-friendly way that will fit comfortably onto your child's bookshelf.
Mummy's Lump is available from your Breast Cancer Care nurse or online at www.ashleycharitabletrust.org.uk

## Support Available

### CLAN – Cancer Link Aberdeen and North

CLAN is an independent charity for anyone affected by any type of cancer at any time from diagnosis onwards. Whether affected personally, as a carer, family member or close friend, CLAN's services are available to anyone affected by cancer. Clan House, Caroline Place, Aberdeen, AB25 2TH
Tel: 01224-647000 enquiries@clanhouse.org

## Helping young people

Clan House also supports youngsters affected by cancer, whether they are the patient, a relative or a friend. Support workers for children and young people offer a confidential service which will

- Provide information
- Listen to the child or young person
- Allow the child or young person to explore difficult feelings in a safe and secure environment
- Bereavement work

Support can be offered on an individual basis or in groups at CLAN House, at home or elsewhere (eg at school). For enquiries, please call 01224-651033 or email Support@clanhouse.org.

There is also a Children's Group (for children affected by cancer) that meets monthly for a range of activities. My own children have been to workshops, performances, craft sessions and sports, giving them the chance to speak to other adults and children if they wish, or enjoy a bit of fun time away from the problems of cancer. Contact Clan House Children's Group on 01224-647000.

Other areas have Maggie Centres or equivalent. See www.maggiescentres.org for information.

# Be Breast Aware

The future for breast cancer is positive with early diagnosis, new treatments and further research being invaluable. Breast Care Nurse Val Bain gives an idea of what to look for:

**How to be Breast Aware:**
- Look at your breasts in the mirror with your arms by your side and then raised behind the head
- Look at your breasts while placing hands on hips and pressing inwards until chest muscles tighten
- Look from every angle
- Feel your breasts at a convenient time eg in the shower or bath with soapy hands, or when dressing or lying on the bed
- Feel all parts of the breasts with the flat of fingers gently and firmly, not squeezing or prodding
- Feel behind the nipple and then up into the armpit, paying particular attention to the upper outer quarter of the chest
- Feel for any lump or thickening in the breast or armpit. Look and feel for anything that is new for you.

**Changes to look for:**
- A lump or thickening which is different to the rest of the breast tissue
- A nipple becomes inverted, changes shape or position
- Discharge from one or both nipples
- Skin changes including puckering or dimpling
- Swelling under the armpit or around the collar bone
- One breast becomes larger or lower
- A rash on or around the nipple

**And finally, remember the five-point code:**
1. Know what is normal for you
2. Look and feel
3. Know what changes to look for
4. Attend breast screening if aged 50 or over
5. REPORT ANY CHANGES WITHOUT DELAY

**Breast Cancer Care** is the UK's leading provider of information, practical assistance and emotional support for anyone affected by **Breast Cancer.** Find out more on the website www.breastcancercare.org.uk or www.breastcancercare.co.uk

**Macmillan Cancer Support** improves the lives of people affected by cancer by providing provide practical, medical and financial support and pushing for better cancer care. Find out more on www.macmillan.org

For more information about the **Bling Fling** or to donate to the **Bling Fling Charities,** please look up the website on www.blingfling.org or contact the Bling Fling team on enquiries@blingfling.org

# With thanks to:

Prof S Heys, to whom I owe my life; Val Bain, whose support and optimism kept me focused and sane throughout my journey; my husband Graham Read, who let me fight my battle my way while working hard to give me a secure base to fight from; my children Matthew and Emma who kept life normal and continue to make me proud by their positive approach to life; my parents for always being there and for giving me a place to cry and a shoulder to cry on; my sisters Heidi and Erica and brother Keith and their families for their love and non-judgemental friendship; the Read family – and especially Skerry - for sharing our burden in the early days and supporting us through the darkest times; the girls from the Bling Fling committee – Janine, Lesley, Lisa, Pam and Lorraine - who provided the laughs, support and many wonderful memories which have made this year extra special; Sandy who always makes me smile and whose crazy outlook on life makes me feel like the sane one; Fiona, my oldest and dearest friend who has always been an absolute rock when I needed it most; Gavin and Susan who have had their own annus horribilus and were still there for me throughout mine; Ian who kept the door open for me to return to my interests when the time was right; to my counsellor, who handed me back the strings of my life and helped me to fly again when the battle was over, and to my other many wonderful friends, both old, new and rekindled during the past year – from Aberdeen Royal Hospitals Trust, Clan, Aberdeen Gang Show, the Evening Express, Book Group, Ante Natal Class, neighbours, theatre groups, school and college friends, Facebook chums - and anyone who has sent me a card or texted me to say they were thinking of me. Every one of you has played your own special role in my life and journey, and I couldn't have gone through the last year without you... thank you.

# Book Group Questions

**Doing It With Bling On writer Sonja Rasmussen is a keen Book Group member, and found great comfort from her fellow bookies while going through cancer treatment. Many of these questions are based on their feedback on her book.**

Did Doing It With Bling On fulfil your expectations? In what ways?

"I'm normally a very slow reader but I read, and read, and read. It really was compulsive reading for me." Did you read it very quickly – why do you think it was so readable. Was it beneficial to read it in one sitting?

"Your idea of including texts is a very clever and honest way of keeping your story even more immediate and real." What did you think of the use of texts? Did you think the memoir style worked or did it jump around too much for you?

Was it worthwhile including other people's stories and interviews? What did they add to the book?

Someone said this book made her realise how lonely a journey it was going through cancer treatment. Do you get a feeling of isolation at any point from the book?

Several times in the book Sonja refers to herself as being 'lucky'. This feeling was planted right at the beginning when Janine said 'You'll be one of the lucky ones who will appreciate your life far more once this is all over'. Do you agree that anyone diagnosed with cancer is lucky – and has that view changed now?

What about the Bling Fling story. How important was that to the book, and to Sonja's breast cancer journey?

Sonja used clothing and make-up to disguise the fact that she was going through something huge... how much do you think women do that anyway?

The colour red is important to this story... red hair, red nails.... there is also a lot of focus on clothes at certain points. Why do you think Sonja remembers what she was wearing in such detail?

"Your story brought me to tears as many times as it made me chuckle". Do you agree that Sonja's story made you laugh and cry in equal measure? What was the overabiding mood of the book for you – upbeat or tear-jerking?

Did it surprise you where the real lows were to be found – and the real highs. For instance, the first chemotherapy trip and operation were portrayed as highlights in the book – is that expected?

Which of the people involved in Sonja's story make most impact when you're reading?

"I'm glad you mentioned Audrey especially in the way you did as a very positive person and the randomness of cancer and responding to treatment". Sonja hoped Audrey's story would make an impact on the reader in the same way that Audrey had made an impact on her. Do you think she succeeded?

Did it strike you as you were reading that Sonja's story is like that of any other woman going through a crisis?

How important was the part Sonja's children played in the book – and in her journey - do you think?

"No wonder you're a journalist, you see so much, and write about it with such endearing openness. I love how you especially see the comical side of life!" Do you think Sonja's journalistic background is evident in her book? In what way has the fact that she is a journalist helped or hindered the writing?

"I read it over 2 nights, the first night I cried quite a lot, found it very emotional. The second half of book, I found more informative, particularly comments from professionals." Sonja wrote the book in two sittings – the first as therapy for herself soon after the Bling Fling, and the second further down the road of recovery, so it was more planned and thought through rather than spontaneous. Can you tell the difference in styles, and does it work that way?

Towards the end of the book, Janine said: "I'd never thought until you came through this what a massive hurdle it is to recover from cancer. Now you probably have 40 years ahead of you like the rest of us, but you also have the experience of having seen your mortality. I don't know how I would cope with that." Had that ever crossed your mind before? Has this book made you think differently about anything?

People's reactions to the book have been different – one reader said when she finished she felt totally and emotionally drained. Another said it was a wonderful story of strength, and friendship. How did you feel when you finished reading? What has stuck with you from the book? What are your lasting impressions?

"This book is "bottled inspiration"...brilliant." So says Prof Heys... In what way is it inspiring?

"Expect lots of ripples on the pond from this book." In what way will professionals learn from Sonja's book? In what ways could it change the views of people about breast cancer treatment?